28 DAY
Reframe

Shift Your Perception
Heal Your Emotions
Change Your Life

KEELY STEELE THOMAS

Table of Contents

Part I

Welcome!

Thank you so much for joining the 28 Day Reframe Community and for being committed to your own well-being. We must love ourselves enough to take the steps required to heal negative emotions that are barriers to our futures and successes. Here's the deal though, most people you know will not take the steps required to clear their paths. This makes you unique!

I am so proud of you and happy for you!

Please remember that not everyone will appreciate your decision to find healing. Not everyone will appreciate the healing you work toward or the changes you make as a result. You might even find your circle of friends changing. It's okay to let the people who are unhappy about the positive changes go. Accept the changes, assume they are for the best and seek to surround yourself with people who are positive and kind. Choose people who will encourage you to be the very best version of you who are.

Now, back to you. Here's the deal, working through your negative emotions will free you to love yourself more and to love others more completely. Working on ourselves does not give us a license to be selfish but it gives us permission to take good care of ourselves. Taking good care of yourself will then increase your capacity to influence and bless the world around you. It's really a win for you, a win for those around you, and a win for the world.

Some of you lean toward selfishness and self-absorption (please don't take this as a judgement – keep reading) and I'm of the opinion that you are that way because you have not found freedom yet. This is your first step in the direction of freedom and a greater capacity to be a blessing to those around you. Congratulations! I promise on the other side of this you'll love that you let go of having the world revolve around you. Hard to imagine right now, but your quality of life will greatly improve.

Some of you lean more toward extreme selflessness. In your world, everyone else comes first. You are almost always last. Please don't think that by doing all this work that you will suddenly become a selfish person. You will not. The work that you do will only prove to help you serve all those people that you love so much in a healthier way. Their lives will improve and so will yours.

Why this process? Well, here's what I've found. As a culture, we've fallen in love with our own personal stories. We love them more than we love our possible futures. We love them more than we love healing. We love the story more than we love ourselves. We love our story more than we love the friends and family we are blessed to have. We want to hold onto the stories tightly. Don't get me wrong, your story is important. It has shaped you into who you are – for good and for bad. But what if we didn't feel the need to live in our past story any longer? What if we could move past the old story? It doesn't go away, but we can loosen our grip on the story enough to find healing and a brighter, much healthier future story.

I'm a huge fan of counseling. My amazing, wise mom put me in counseling when I was in the fifth grade and over the years I've seen different types of counselors at various times in my life. Most of them have been wonderfully helpful. However, often times, the sessions were just my telling the same stories that I had told hundreds of times complete with buckets of tears. I was truly in pain and yet not finding healing. I knew I was missing something.

What was I missing? Probably a lot of things. Ha! I've been on a journey of figuring that out for well over a decade. Just sitting here thinking about where I've come blows me away. I'm going to share with you all that I've discovered. I'm trusting that you will trust me, work through the exercises, and find not just healing, but tools for facing challenges in the future.

I'm a practical woman. I want answers to problems to be simple and straight forward. I avoid fluff and drama, if possible, so my goal for these 28 Days is simplicity and practicality. Know that I'd love to support you in person, but I hope that I will be able to help you support and encourage yourself during this process by providing the steps to take and a new set of tools to appropriately handle the challenges in your future. I'm for you!

What can you expect?

I've designed this program after working with people one-on-one. It's a similar process to what I walk people through in person. I can't be there to talk you through this, but I can share what I've learned with you and believe that you can be helped as much as someone who would sit in my office.

Walking through these 28 Days' worth of assignments will be as close as we can get to sitting with me in my office. Take one day at a time, following the assignment closely. Do not make this complicated. Just follow the assignment as given. Now is not the time to relive every pain you've experienced. You don't have to relive it to experience healing. You also don't have to deny the pain in hopes that it will go away, but I'm trusting that if you are here then you are done with denial.

This process will take some discipline on your part but be encouraged knowing that some days will take only ten minutes. That's not much time at all. We all waste more time than that on social media. Right? If you miss a day, don't panic, or get discouraged. Just pick up where you left off and keep going. In fact, life happens, so I realize that you most likely will, on occasion, miss a day. And sometimes you'll need a little time to breathe because an assignment hit you a little hard. That's okay, my friend. Just take a day or two to breathe and then jump back in where you left off.

Some assignments will be simple for you and some will be more difficult. On the simple days, take it seriously but just be thankful for the fact that particular assignment isn't very challenging. Of course, some days will be challenging. On those days, take good care of yourself and don't allow yourself to be dragged down by the past. You can face it, forgive it, and let it go. Trust me, I'm not glossing over the hurts and the pains, I'm just ready for you to be free of them. All the assignments are critical, the easy ones as well as the difficult. When you get to the end of the 28 Days, each of the days will make sense to you. You will see how the puzzle fits together. You'll understand how each of the pieces play a role in your healing.

It took me five years to really put all of this together, but you get to do it in 28 Days. Then you get to use what you've learned for the future, because there will be more hurts, more pain, more challenges because life happens, and we are surrounded by humans. The tools you learn during this time will serve you well when those challenging times come. These tools will enable you to have a brighter future, more success in business or your career, better relationships, and a greater capacity for giving and receiving love.

This will be one of the greatest decisions you've ever made. Get mentally prepared for the work. Expect greatness. Expect healing. Expect joy. Expect peace. Expect FREEDOM.

Why?

Negative emotions can be a huge barrier to success and growth in life. Careers, relationships, spiritual growth, processes of the brain, and physical health can all be hindered by negative emotions. If one of those is being hindered, then you can assume that others are being hindered as well. And, you may not even be aware that these areas of your life are being affected. It may not be obvious to you.

I had a client who was great at interacting with people on just an occasional basis, but as her relationships deepened, she couldn't handle the intimacy. Her negative emotions were getting in the way of having close relationships with family as well as friends. She couldn't see it and didn't understand why relationships were falling apart. However, as she worked through her challenges and found healing, she found that she had the capacity to allow people she loved to get closer to her.

Another client struggled to keep a job. It's not that he wasn't capable of doing the job or that he wasn't qualified for the positions. However, he had trauma as a young child that caused him to close off his heart. Instead of being in touch with his emotional side, he became extremely analytical. He just couldn't connect with others and was abrasive without being aware of his cold manner of dealing with people. He didn't want to be abrasive, but he didn't know how to be any other way. He's still on his journey of healing and finding ways to connect to his heart, but he is growing and now can see how his behavior affects those around him.

After my daughter was born in 2006, I was so ill that I spent most of my day in bed. With two small children to take care of, obviously, this was unacceptable. As I began to rebuild my body with vitamins, minerals, homeopathy, and herbs, I began to get stronger and find physical healing. However, there were some physical challenges that just weren't being taken care of no matter how committed I was to do all it took to tackle those challenges. A wonderful friend told me that I needed emotional healing to truly find physical healing. He jump-started this journey and I'll be forever grateful. My husband and I were both truly amazed at the changes we saw as I took steps toward healing. It was a journey that took time and effort on my part, but with each step I took, emotional and physical healing followed.

The negative emotions I was carrying around had settled in different parts of my body. This is true for all of us. You see, emotions have frequencies just like everything in our world has a frequency. These frequencies can be for our benefit or for our harm. Positive emotions have vibrations that bring health and healing while negative emotions have vibrations that bring sickness and pain.

Negative emotions can also negatively affect the processes of the brain. Dr. Caroline Leaf is a great resource for more research in this area. Dr. Leaf is a cognitive neuroscientist with a PhD in Communication Pathology specializing in Neuropsychology. Her research on how negative thoughts affect how we communicate and behave is powerful. In fact, she has been on the cutting edge of the research of how changes in our mind can affect the brain's ability to change and even develop further. We all would enjoy what I call greater brain capacity, right? I want my brain to function at its highest ability, so I continue to work toward healing and positive thoughts and emotions.

Your Personal Motivation

First, it is imperative that you have a journal or notebook to work through all the exercises. It will be encouraging to look back at all your work and see the progress you've made.

Take some time to think through why you have chosen to seek out healing and freedom. It's always good to know the why behind what you are doing so that you can keep reminding yourself as you walk along the journey. Some of you are here because of a physical illness, knowing that as your emotions are healed your body will have the capacity to heal as well. Those negative emotions won't get in the way, any longer, to complete wellness. Some of you know that the negative emotions are getting in the way of your success in different areas of life. Who wouldn't want to make more money? Do you want a raise? Do you want more clients for your business? Clearing out negative thoughts will clear out negative patterns. Business relationships will improve. Your capacity for creativity and planning will improve. Are the negative emotions preventing you from closer personal relationships? Loving, close relationships are a great "why". And, some of you are so tired of feeling hurt, sadness, anger, and frustration all the time. Joy, peace, and love are amazing "whys".

Whatever your motivation, just keep it in mind so that you can stay motivated. Let me encourage you to write down why you want to start on this journey in your new journal or notebook so that you'll keep putting one foot in front of the other when life gets busy or this process becomes intense.

We all need reminders. Set yourself up for success and find ways to remind yourself of all that you want to achieve during these 28 Days. Sprinkle a reminder of your "why" throughout your personal calendar. When you come to the end of the 28 Days, you'll feel such a great sense of achievement for having accomplished all you set out to achieve.

Why are you on this journey?

Take Care

While you are walking through this process, I want you to take really good care of yourself. Your mind and your body need support. Your mind is affected by all that is going on with your body. So, water, food, sunshine, exercise, deep breathing, and sleep are going to be of utmost importance over the next 28 Days. It's only 28 Days. You can do anything for 28 Days!

There are two things you need to think through about water. First is making sure that you are drinking enough water each and every day. A good rule of thumb is to drink half of your body weight in ounces of water every single day. So, if you weigh 200 pounds, then you'll need to drink 100 ounces throughout the day. If you drink coffee, soda, green tea, or black tea, then it is important to add in more water. If you have an 8-ounce cup of coffee, then you'll need to add in another 8 ounces of water. So, the 200-pound person who drinks one cup of coffee each day will now need to take in 108 ounces of water each and every day.

I have a couple of tricks that I like to use to help me get in all of my ounces in a day. Measuring out your ounces in the morning can help or purchasing a large cup with a straw that you will refill throughout the day. I have one that holds 32 ounces, so I don't have to refill a million times. Using a straw can help you to take in water more quickly. People who drink through a straw tend to drink more. Setting a timer for 15 minutes and then making sure that you drink a few ounces each time the timer goes off is another trick to help you stay hydrated.

The second thing I hope you'll consider is getting a good water filtration system. Research what is really in our tap water and you'll be surprised (possibly a little appalled). We use a Berkey water filter in our home. We have two sizes and our recommendation is that you get the largest size available. After using water to fill a pot for pasta, wash vegetables, fill glass water bottles, fill sports jugs, and then just normal drinking, we have found that the smaller one just doesn't meet all of our needs as a family of four. You can go to www.reframecenter.com to learn more if you don't already have what you need.

You also need to make sure you are getting proper nutrition. It is so easy to just stop by the local fast food restaurant to pick something up for dinner, but is that really the best option for your body during this time? I'm going to go with probably not. Instead do a little prep work and you'll be so glad you did. Some of you are already good at eating well and so I'm not talking to you. I want to talk to those of you who think that eating well is just too much work.

Every week stock up on those organic salads at the grocery store that are in a bag, ready to go. They aren't my favorite option, but they are MUCH better than stopping at fast food. You just have to open it up, empty it into a big bowl and then dump the other contents of the bag into the salad. Top it with the salad dressing that is provided, and you are good to go. Now, I don't want to get letters about this. Yes, there are even better options out there, but we are addressing the convenience issues right now for those who are tired at the end of the day and are used to stopping by restaurants and picking up dinner.

Do you own a slow cooker? It can be your best friend! When you have dinner done at 7:00 in the morning because all your ingredients are in your slow cooker and you've remembered to turn it on, well, it's just the best feeling in the world. When you get home from work, there is dinner smelling yummy and ready to feed you, your family, and friends. Notice that you didn't have to stop by the local fast food on that night. Win! And, if you have leftovers, then you can have those for lunch the next day or find another way to serve that meal for dinner the next night or two nights from now. If I make a roast and I have leftovers, then two nights from now I can take that meat and make yummy sandwiches out of it. I'll add a salad and we're all pretty happy.

I keep a list on my phone of our favorite dinners, so that when I'm trying to plan or running by the grocery store, I don't have to think too much about what we are going to do for dinners for the week.

For myself, I've found that focusing on eating eggs, meat, and veggies gives me the best energy and focus that I need for my day. Please do some research and decide what works best for you. Keeping sugar out of your diet is always a good idea. Now, don't think that my crew and I eat perfectly all the time. We don't, but we are constantly working toward eating better and finding convenient ways to get the best nutrition in our diets.

I like to make things in large batches on the weekends. I'll make gluten-free pancakes made with gluten free flour and lots of eggs, so they have tons of protein, put them in a container in the refrigerator or freezer and then just heat them up throughout the week for breakfast. We'll eat some chicken sausage or beef bacon with it, and we are good to go. They also make good snacks. Breakfast tacos are also a hit. We don't do those as often because we try to eat low gluten, but if I make them in bulk, then I can just wrap them refrigerator up individually and put them in the freezer. Before bed, I'll move some of the burritos to the to thaw overnight and then just throw them in the oven to heat up while we all get ready in the morning. Super simple.

Another cook ahead trick is to grill a lot of different meats on the weekend so that you have meats prepared for all meals throughout the week. You can grill hamburger patties, chicken, sausage, steak, and any other meats that your family enjoys and have them ready to reheat in the oven for your meals.

Now, for lunch there are a million options. There are some really good, healthy restaurants out there, so make good decisions when you eat out. However, the bag salad with last night's leftover chicken is just too easy, healthy, and inexpensive. Hard to pass that up. Hummus with crackers (Nut Thins are our favorites), a wrap you made at home in less than five minutes, some pecans, a piece of fruit, and some coconut milk yogurt are all simple, easy solutions.

Your body needs to be strong during these 28 Days, because your emotions do affect your body and the food you put in your body affects your emotions. So, please love yourself enough to support your body with healthy choices during this time.

Oh, now one of my favorite subjects, sunshine! How do you feel when you are sitting out in the sun for ten minutes? Do you feel your mood lift? Do you feel stronger and more capable? Do you feel relaxed and less stressed? I know I do! I just so enjoy the sun and the way it makes me feel. Also, our bodies produce vitamin D when we spend time in the sun. In the past I dealt with depression from a vitamin D deficiency, so you can imagine that I make sure that I don't get deficient in vitamin D any longer. The Vitamin D Council (https://www.vitamindcouncil.org/about-vitamin-d/) is a great resource for information about Vitamin D.

Now for my encouragement for you to exercise at least three days a week. No, you don't have to join a gym or start doing some intense workout. Walking around the block for 15 minutes can truly make a huge difference in the way your body and mind function. Is the weather bad? Do some exercises while you watch a movie or listen to a book. Please find something you enjoy. You are much more likely to exercise consistently if you are doing something that is fun and feels good to you. My husband, Brian, is a runner. That man loves to run. It's really not my favorite activity, but I love spending time on the recumbent, stationary bicycle. In fact, I love it so much that frequently I'll decided that I'm going to ride for 20 minutes and then find myself riding for an hour. I'll watch a movie, read a book, catch up on a favorite show, listen to a podcast, or chat with a friend on the phone (if I'm going at a leisurely pace). Just find what works for you, not for someone else.

The internet also makes it really easy to find exercises that we like. There are thousands of great (and free) exercise videos and apps out there. YouTube really has made this more fun for me. Search different key words to find just what you are looking for. The variety of stretching, weightlifting, low-impact, high-impact, and dance exercise videos out there is phenomenal.

Unless we are in the middle of cardio exercise, most of us spend our day breathing with only 10% capacity of our lungs. Breathing deeply helps to lower stress among other things. Right now, we'll just focus on the lowering of stress since our next 28 Days are going to be a journey toward healing. Every day I want you to pause to focus on your breathing. Just one minute a day can make a huge impact but think about how that would be multiplied if you focused on your breathing every hour. The easiest thing to do it to stop every hour on the hour to breathe deeply.

So, here's a simple, easy to remember exercise. You are going to take a slow, deep breath in through your nose making your belly rise (not your chest). Do that while counting to seven in your head. Then hold that breath while you count to four. Then again, count to seven while you slowly breathe out of your mouth. Just think, 7-4-7. Repeat this breathing exercise for one minute.

When you are taking that slow, deep breath in, be sure that your belly is going out. This is how you know that you are getting air into the lowest part of your lungs. I also like to do this when I get in bed at night. The deep breathing will take your mind off of the troubles of your day or the worries of tomorrow. This will also relax you and get your body ready for sleep.

You also need to make sure that you are getting good sleep at night. We're all different here. My husband doesn't require as much sleep as I do. I really function well when I've had seven to nine hours of sleep. He can function on six to seven hours. Think about how much sleep you need and make that happen. Do not stay up late watching TV or scrolling through Facebook, Twitter, and Instagram. Get to bed early and build in time for you to fall asleep. When Brian's head hits the pillow, I can count to ten and he'll be asleep before I actually finish counting. I, on the other hand, take a little more time to fall asleep. This can take me anywhere from five to thirty minutes. So, I build in time for me to process my day and pray. The counting of hours of sleep doesn't start until I actually fall asleep.

Turn your phone off at night or at least move it out of your room or across the room. Cell phones can negatively affect sleep, so get it away from you. Turn your Wi-Fi off every night at the router before you go to sleep as well. You don't need it while you sleep. Make sure your room is nice and dark. Even the dimmest of light can stop the body's production of melatonin. Get comfortable. How do you like your covers? What do you like to sleep in? What temperature works best for you? Make those things happen. Set the stage for a great night of sleep. Make sleep a priority! Every part of your body as well as your mind functions better with consistent, deep sleep.

The goal here is keeping your body strong while you are releasing negative emotions. The stronger and healthier your body is, the healthier and stronger your mind will be also. You will be able to think more clearly and make better decisions for your life. Let's take a holistic approach to your emotional healing. Support your whole self during this process.

Bach Flowers

Have you heard of Bach Flowers? I hadn't until 2007 and now am grateful to have them at my disposal. There are 38 Bach Flower Remedies that were discovered and researched by Dr. Edward Bach in the 1920s and 1930s. You can find these Bach Flower Remedies at any health food or supplement store. Each remedy correlates with a fundamental emotion. Honeysuckle is great for someone who is stuck living in the past, while Aspen is selected when someone has an unknown fear. These 38 Bach Flower Remedies are worth your further research, because as Dr. Bach said, "they are able, like beautiful music, or any gloriously uplifting thing which gives us inspiration, to raise our very natures, and bring us nearer to our Souls: and by that very act, to bring us peace, and relieve our sufferings."

The Bach Flower bottles give descriptions about the flowers, so you choose which one you think is best for you. Muscle testing for the Bach Flowers is another option if you know how to do that.

Group Work

I love the idea of getting a group of people together that you trust to walk through this process with. Make sure that it is a safe group of people and that they will hold you accountable to pursuing healing. However, I would say that you need to put some rules into place, because I've found that when you get a group of hurting people together it frequently can turn into a misery loves company club. The group can become a forum for just telling our stories over and over again. We think this will bring healing, because if we could just find some compassion then maybe it would all go away. If we could just find the right person to love us enough, then we'd find healing. However, you won't find healing in any of these people. Use it as an accountability group and it's a good idea.

Guidelines

1. Let go of your love affair with your story.
2. Don't expect that others will fall in love with your story.
3. Make sure that you aren't monopolizing the group's time.
4. Focus on finding forgiveness and healing.
5. Focus on the steps you are taking to support yourself in the process.
6. Focus on sharing affirmations.
7. Encourage each other to keep speaking forgiveness.
8. Share victories.
9. Share hope.
10. Celebrate forgiveness, hope, and freedom as a group.

Start off your time together saying an affirmation together. You can use mine or come up with your own. Remember, it needs to be positive and in the present.

I am healthy and whole, mentally, physically, spiritually, and emotionally.

I choose forgiveness, love, joy, and peace.

I surround myself with people who love, support, and encourage me.

If you are meeting each week, then you can share with one another what you are experiencing as you speak out your affirmations. You can also talk about the work you've done in the previous week. Again, don't give too much back story on the challenges you are working through. The details of the lions are not important. What is important is what you are doing for healing. Support one another in the process, not in the lion stories.

Tell one another the great things you are doing in your lives to support your processes of healing. Share your successes and joys. Share any blocks you might be experiencing in healing and help one another come up with ideas for pushing through those blocks. Most of all, remind each other that this is worth it. Encourage one another to keep going.

Part II

Day 1

Okay, so are you ready to jump in? I know you're ready, so let's go!

The good news is that Day 1 is not a gut-wrenching day. However, this day is critical for setting the stage for the rest of the days. We've got to build a firm foundation to keep you strong for the days to come. This is your opportunity to set yourself up for success for the next 27 days.

I'm a huge believer in the fact that you've got to find a way to be your own biggest support. People may come and go. Your friends and family may not always be available to encourage you or uphold you during a difficult time, so let's figure out ways for you to do that for yourself.

Your assignment is two-fold. First, I want you to make a list of three things that you can do every week that can help meet your encouragement needs. These are not to be complicated.

During one of the most difficult times of my life, I sat down and really figured out what I needed to do to take good care of myself. For me, I needed to have lunch, dinner, or breakfast with one really good friend each and every week. I was faithful to get one friend date on my calendar every week. The great part about this time with my friends was that I had a freedom to vent (make sure that you don't vent the whole time). Laughing with my friends also gave some relief to the intense stress that I was experiencing throughout my week. My friends were also sharing with me about their lives which got my mind off myself. Being able to love on my friends and show them compassion as well pulled my brain out of any repetitive thinking that I was stuck in.

Working out five days a week was imperative, because I needed to burn the emotions that were boiling inside of me. These weren't intense workouts, but they were enough to help me. We talked about this earlier and what is important is that you find something you enjoy. If you don't enjoy it, it is more difficult to be consistent. Exercise increases oxygen to the brain, reduces stress and anxiety, improves your mood, and improves memory. I don't know about you, but all of that makes me want to get up and move my body!

My faith is important to me, so I spent time every day in quiet by myself praying. When I pray, I feel calm and at peace because I've laid down all the worries that I've been carrying around with me. I realize that I'm not in charge of all of life and that I'm only responsible for my actions and responses to life around me. That time allows me to be still and then emerge with less chaos and confusion.

Time with friends, exercise and prayer all grounded me, gave me sanity, and helped me to put one foot in front of the other. So, instead of just being in survival mode (which I could have chosen), I was taking care of myself and thriving in the middle of a challenging time in my life. I was faithful to myself. As you keep commitments to yourself, you will build confidence. I kept these appointments with myself, just like I would keep them with a friend. Loving myself was the key to staying faithful to myself. It was a choice. It is a choice for you as well. What will you choose?

So, sit down and think about what would really support you during this process. Maybe for you it's doing something creative every day, hitting the gym, or calling a friend who lives far away. Taking a long bath once a week may really refuel you. This list is going to be different for each person that does this, so if you are walking through this process with a group of friends, remember that what encourages you won't be the same as what encourages your friend.

The items on your list can be things that you will do daily, weekly, or even several times a week. Make sure it is frequent enough to keep your mental state lifted. Get it on your calendar and take them seriously. Do not skimp on this step. Please, please, please take good care of yourself.

The other criterion for this list is that the items on the list must support you. For instance, please don't choose anything that would provide short-term relief but that could potentially sabotage your long-term goals. Think, really think, what would help, not harm. Be smart here. So, while you might get some short-term relief from multiple beers at your local bar, this may not be the best option for your healing journey. So, make your list of three things you can do consistently that will support you and get them on your calendar.

So, the second half of your assignment for today is to write out an affirmation that you will put on your bathroom mirror, on your phone, in your car and next to your computer. You want this to be something you see multiple times a day. One of my favorite ways to post an affirmation is by putting it in a Ziploc bag and then hanging it in the shower. It's a good use of time. You can shower and encourage yourself at the same time.

Now, there are guidelines to this affirmation. It needs to be in the present and in the positive. So, let's look at some examples of what NOT to do:

> I will not spend my time obsessing over these situations any longer.

That statement is negative and is not in the present. Please do not do an affirmation like this. It isn't really affirming, is it?

> I am no longer obsessing over my hurts any longer.

That is in the present, but it is still negative. It is focusing on what you don't want rather on what you do want and what you are looking forward to.

Feel free to use my affirmation if you'd rather. I've made sure that it is both positive and present. This type of affirmation can give you the personal support you need to walk through this 28 Day challenge.

I am healthy and whole, mentally, physically, spiritually, and emotionally.
I choose forgiveness, love, joy, and peace.
I surround myself with people who love, support, and encourage me.
I deserve to be healthy, whole, joyful, peaceful, and loved.

I need you to speak this affirmation *out loud* at least twice a day every single day for the next 28 Days. Why out loud? There is an amazing connection between our voice and our bodies. So, when you say your affirmation out loud it makes a huge impact on your emotions, your body, and your mind. You'll have to trust me on this one. After you've done this for several days, you'll become a believer.

So, write out your affirmation and post it at least on your bathroom mirror. Get to work, remember that your future self is counting on you, and let's meet back again tomorrow for Day 2.

"The secret of getting ahead is getting started." Mark Twain

Day 2

Hey! Welcome to Day 2! I hope you enjoyed walking through the ways you can support yourself during this process on Day 1. It's all about setting your future self up for success. And, that affirmation you wrote yesterday can make all the difference in your mental state during your journey. Keeping positive thoughts flowing through your mind will prevent your getting bogged down in the negative emotions that we will be tackling.

Ready for your assignment today? Of course you are! You are here!

"Believe in yourself! Have faith in your abilities! Without a humble but reasonable confidence in your own powers you cannot be successful or happy." Norman Vincent Peale

Today I need to you make a timeline of your life. Don't get overwhelmed, this is going to be easier than it sounds. Draw a straight line across your paper. Your birth will be on the left of your line and present day will be on the right. Above that line I want you to place ten major events in your life that have been positive. Then, below the line you'll place ten major events in your life that have been negative.

I don't want you to feel confined to ten events, so if you come up with more than ten then that's okay with me. However, I don't want you to do more than fifteen because I don't want you to get too deep in the events. You'll have assignments, in the future, with these events and if they aren't narrowed down, then the future assignments could be more challenging.

Some of your positive and negative will be life events like births, deaths, graduations while others will be challenges, hurts, and more painful events. On my timeline, I have the births of my children as positive events in my life and the death of my mom as a major negative event in my life. Those are regular life events. I also have some hurtful events on my timeline when people hurt me, some intentionally and some unintentionally. I expect that you will have events that fit into both the regular life events category and in the hurt-by-people category.

Get to work and remember that your work will pay off as you walk through these assignments. You are building a better life and a better future. I'm so proud of you for moving forward and doing what it takes to find healing and wellness in all areas of your life. You are worth it!

By the way, if you are going through this process with other people, be discerning. Sometimes we can inadvertently share our journey with people who either don't really care or who will actually use this information against us. I discovered once that a woman I had shared deeply with could not actually be trusted. Or it could possibly be that she could be trusted during a previous period of my life but can now no longer be trusted. We need to assess our relationships and really be prudent.

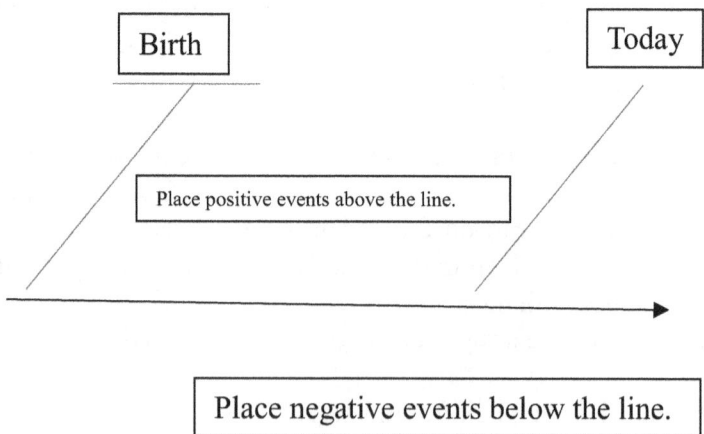

| Birth | | Today |

Place positive events above the line.

Place negative events below the line.

"It is in your moments of decision that your destiny is shaped."
Tony Robbins

Day 3

I'd love to be sitting across from you right now. I'd love to look at your timeline and ask you questions about the events and situations that you put above and below the line. I'd love to just dive in a little deeper with you to find out more. You are a unique person with unique gifts and talents whose life has been blessed in many ways and hurt in many ways. Your story is a one of a kind and I'd love to be able to hear it. Be sure to let safe people into your life so they can hear your story. And you, in turn, can dive into the lives of those around you. The effort and time are so worth it as long as you are making wise choices in your relationships.

Today is a thankfulness day. You are going to spend time speaking, *out loud*, thankfulness about each of those items above the line. Take them one by one. Take time doing this. Be specific. For instance, if you are thankful for a particular job you got then speak thankfulness about the job, the people you work for and with, the parts of the job that you really enjoy, the knowledge you have gained from the job, the financial aspect of the job, the work environment, and anything else you can think of.

Looking at your items from all angles can give you a deeper appreciation. Again, speaking *out loud* connects all of you to that thankfulness. Your body, your spirit, and your soul will all feel the thankfulness and joy will overflow.

Soak it in even if you aren't a big feeler. Use this time to further build your mind and body. You are building new roads in your mind. The new roads in your mind will positively affect your emotions and your body. This takes time, effort, and energy, but it will be worth it in the long run.

You will get out of this what you put into it. Love yourself enough to do it and do it well. If you have surrounded yourself with negative people, they may be taken back by your newfound joy and thankfulness. Don't worry. They will either join you in the new attitude or you'll start to attract people who are full of joy. That sounds pretty amazing, doesn't it? Enjoy this day and let's meet back here tomorrow for more.

Write down some of the details of all you are feeling thankful for in your journal so you can come back and revisit what you spoke thankfulness about.

Day 4

I hope you really enjoyed speaking thankfulness for the items above your line. Remember how that feels. Remember the smiles you felt on the inside. When tough days come, and they will, then go back to finding things to be thankful for and remember those that you are already thankful for. Speak *out loud* to encourage your whole self. Continue to live life intentionally thankful.

Your assignment today is to assess the items below the line. Let's find out which items truly aren't healed yet. Many years ago, I was really struggling with trying to figure out which things in my life were healed and which weren't. I think the struggle came from still having all the memories. We have to keep in mind that, for most of us, we will always remember the circumstances. However, that doesn't mean that those circumstances aren't healed. Maybe they are and maybe they aren't.

During the time that I was working through some hurts, I was being told by a mentor that I still had deep wounds that were affecting me. She named the ones she thought were having the largest negative impact in my life. Funny thing was that I chose, at the time, to believe her rather than assess for myself. Looking back on it, she was completely wrong about which hurts in my life weren't healed. For whatever reason I trusted her more than I trusted myself. As a result, I spent time and energy focusing on circumstances in my life that were really no longer making a huge impact on me. Her suggestion that these hurts were major made them major in my mind. That all changed one day. Instead of letting someone else try to figure out what was going on inside of my heart and my head, I took the time to assess for myself.

I thought through the events in my life from two different perspectives. Were each of these events just annoying houseflies? You know, one gets into your house and flies around annoying you. Then, you don't see it for a while. It's just an annoyance. Or is the event you are assessing a lion? It's crouching in the bush waiting just to overtake you, tackle you, and then eat you alive. You know it's there and your emotions are intense.

These questions changed my life dramatically. I now have my own assessment tools. There is no longer the need to let someone else determine which are truly problems that have not been healed. There are no doubts in my head about what has been healed and what hasn't.

So, I want you to take the assessment tool and assess the items below your line. You are going to spend a short period of time thinking about each individual item. Is your first item a fly or a lion? See how you feel when you think about it. How much emotion comes up for you? Is it annoying or is it going to devour you? Let's not live in denial. If you can't come up with a lion, you might be fooling yourself.

As you assess each item below the line on your timeline, I want you to write fly or lion next to each one.

After you have done that, I want you to pick three of the items you wrote lion next to. Just pick three and circle them. These will be the three we work through during our time together.

My hope is that having a tool to assess what needs to be worked on will give you some relief. I know I felt so much better just knowing that the difficult circumstances that had happened in my life weren't all forever going to remain unhealed. Being able to assess by lion or fly showed me that some had already been healed. What a relief!!!! Remember, the mentor in my life was wrong about the events in my life that needed to be healed. So, don't always just trust that someone else knows. Other people can be helpful, but no one else is inside your head or heart.

My question for you today is: Are you speaking your affirmation out loud at least twice a day? If this is on your bathroom mirror, then just say it immediately after you brush your teeth in the morning and at night before you go to bed. It takes so little time and yet makes such a big impact.

See you tomorrow!

There's only one corner of the universe you can be certain of improving, and that's your own self. – Aldous Huxley

Day 5

Yesterday you assessed your items below the line. You determined which were flies and which were lions. I so hope that was as helpful to you as it was for me. You also picked three of the lions that we will work on together.

Today you are going to pick one of your three lions. Some of you will pick the one that seems the most difficult to you and some will pick the easiest. It is completely up to you as to which one you pick. I want you to feel comfortable with this entire process. We'll call this first situation Lion #1.

Today's assignment is a simple task, but an important one. We are setting the stage for healing. You are going to make a list of all the people involved in Lion #1. I want you to be sure and include yourself in this list. Your name needs to go on this list as you were a part of Lion #1 as well.

Simple, right? Now, for those of you who are feelers, don't get bogged down in the event. This is a simple list – there is no room for rumination in this process. Just get the names down on paper.

Okay, I'm proud of you for sticking with this process and investing in your emotional well-being. This well-being will spread into all areas of your life.

Speak your affirmations! Blessings!

Keep your face always toward the sunshine - and shadows will fall behind you. Walt Whitman

Day 6

"Always do your best. What you plant now, you will harvest later." Og Mandino

I love this quote by Og Mandino. KNOW that all of your work that you are doing now will provide a harvest of healing, joy, and love. Well done!

Yesterday you made a list of all the people involved in Lion #1 and I'm proud of you for taking that step. It may not feel like a big step, but it's an important one.

Today is forgiveness day. This is a great day! Here is where your world begins to be reframed. Oh, I can already hear some shifting in chairs, some clearing of throats, and some arguments coming on. So, let's work through those for a moment.

I find people often fall into one of two categories. Let's examine the first category. These are the people who feel like it is unjust to forgive, like the perpetrator will never get what is coming to them if they do forgive. They believe that holding onto unforgiveness is justified because the person must pay for the hurt inflicted.

I encounter these people frequently and I understand where they are coming from. They are lovers of justice, and I can relate to the love of justice. Let's think through this one for a minute though. Is the other person really being punished because I've determined that I will not forgive them? The answer to that is a resounding "no". That person may not even have any clue that I have chosen to not forgive them. If they do know, is it really affecting them in any way? Probably not. They are going about their lives without any thought of me.

So, let's let go of the idea that we are serving justice by not forgiving someone.

What I want you to do each time you decide to not forgive someone is to picture that person as a boulder right smack dab in the middle of your path on your journey. You have chosen to put that person there. They are not choosing to be there. You are choosing to keep them there. No matter how hard you try to make progress on your path, that boulder keeps getting in the way. You try to climb over it and it just grows. You try to go around it. You try to push it out of the way. Nothing works. The boulder just holds you back and keeps you from reaching your goals.

Forgiveness removes that person from your path and then you no longer have a huge obstacle in your way. I want you to move forward on your journey. How sad would it be to look up when you are 90 years old and have one person be the reason that you didn't achieve your goals, didn't get what you really wanted out of life? And, it wouldn't be their fault, it would be yours. Yikes! I know that's harsh, but it's also true and I care about you enough to say it. The person who hurt you will have forgotten, but if you keep them as an obstacle, then you will have missed out on all that life could be.

I know we've all heard the saying that not forgiving someone is like mixing poison for the person who hurt us and then drinking it ourselves. This is true. Not forgiving someone will fester inside. Picture something rotting deep in your gut and that is a great picture of unforgiveness.

Please keep in mind that forgiveness does not mean that you allow the same hurtful behavior to continue. Nor does it mean that you have to necessarily have that person in your life. As you heal, you will have a greater ability to choose healthy boundary lines in your life.

So, let's give this a shot and see what happens, shall we? Thank you, lovers of justice, for trusting me!

Now, hang there for a minute while I address the too-quick-to-forgive crowd. Now, don't get me wrong, I don't mean that you shouldn't forgive quickly. In fact, please do. However, I know lots of people who say to me, "Oh, I've already forgiven him/her for that." And yet, I can see it all over them that they are still really hurting and holding onto something. They are saying they have forgiven solely because it's the right thing to do. They know they should forgive, so they say they have.

I am a huge believer in speaking things and then having our emotions follow our will. I know this works. I've experienced it and have seen others experience it. However, there is a difference between truly forgiving someone and just glossing over the situation and trying to sweep it to the side. This is going to be a process. This process does not include pretending, denying, or sweeping under the rug. Call the elephant in the room what it is, and you'll find the elephant getting smaller.

Let's begin and see what happens. Remember this is a process. Get all the way through the process and assess what healing has occurred. Today we are going to address each person in Lion #1. I want you to take each person, one by one. Pretend that person is sitting across from you. I want you to say something to that person similar to this:

"_____ (insert that person's name), when you _____ (fill in their part in Lion #1), that really hurt my feelings (or put in what you felt at that time, anger, frustration, sadness, etc.). Today I choose to forgive you, _____ (insert their name) for your part in _____ (Lion #1). I choose to let go of that hurt today. I choose joy and peace right now because I deserve joy and peace."

Go through that exercise with each and every person involved in Lion #1. If there are emotions involved, let them come. Address them. Acknowledge them. Then, let them go by speaking release of them. Give yourself permission to grieve and then give yourself permission to really let go of all the negative emotions.

Please remember that your emotions will follow your will. Today is a day for healing. Choosing to forgive is the launching point for healing and the beginning of your amazing future. Please don't think that I'm trying to gloss over this. It is the <u>beginning</u> of a great process. This is a simple yet also quite complex step. The making of a list is simple. The speaking out loud can be both simple and complex. The working out of emotions is definitely complex. But I want to assure you that the steps you are taking will do the work. Don't make it complicated by over thinking it. Do the work. Be present in the moment. Then watch the healing unfold.

Your name was on the Lion #1 list too, wasn't it? Well then, let's make sure that you speak forgiveness toward yourself as well. Maybe you didn't defend yourself like you wish you had. Maybe you behaved in a way that you just are not happy with. Maybe you said some things that you wish you hadn't said. Insert your name in the forgiveness script.

One last thing about this. If you were too young to have done anything about this situation, then what I want you to do is speak something like this toward yourself:

"_____ (insert your name), when _____ (Lion #1) happened you were not at fault. You were a child and the adults were responsible for taking care of you. This was not your fault. I love you. I do not hold you responsible for what happened."

Sit in that. Really soak in the feeling of being relieved of responsibility for Lion #1. Take a deep breath. Let go of the hurt. Let go of the sadness. Let go of the anger. Keep breathing.

I know that this can be difficult. Some of you may feel immediate relief and healing and that's awesome! Some of you may not feel so great because the emotions are now stirred up and that's perfectly normal. The emotions are normal. Remember that this is a 28 Day process that you are on. There is more to come, and healing awaits. You are worth it!!!! Please hang in there with me and with yourself. This is just the beginning.

I'm on your side cheering for you!

"Accept the challenges so you can feel the exhilaration of victory." George S. Patton

Day 7

Yesterday was a big day and I'm proud of you for pushing through and choosing forgiveness! I'm hoping that you got a good night's rest and are feeling resolute about finishing out the 28 Days. If you are feeling weak and beat down, then just put one foot in front of the other and continue on this journey. Do it because you want a better life, a better thought life, better relationships, a better future.

Today we're going to change our perception of the people involved in Lion #1. I'm not talking about excusing bad behavior or denying events that happened. We are simply reframing the situation to help our minds, emotions, and bodies heal from Lion #1.

I want you to go through your list of people in Lion #1. Ask yourself some questions about each of those people.

-What was going on in that person's life when that situation happened?

-What hurts has that person experienced in the past that may have predisposed them to behave poorly?

-What growth do they need in their life that is making them miss out on the best their life has to offer?

-What hurts is that person inflicting on themselves through their bad behavior?

Asking these questions, again, does not excuse behavior, it simple allows us to see them in a different light and help us to have a greater understanding of and more compassion for them.

This exercise was huge for me. I have a person in my life who hurt me multiple times. It was very painful for me even to think of this person. We'll call this person Lynn. Many years ago, when I was working through my hurts that involved Lynn, I had an amazing experience. I imagined in my mind that Lynn and I were sitting across the table from one another. I felt very uncomfortable because we were sitting too close to one another. So, in my mind I moved us further away from one another. I still felt uncomfortable, so I moved us to a beautiful, wide open field. Then I moved us about 30 feet from one another. I felt much more comfortable in the field, like I could breathe. Then I saw Lynn pull out a gun (like a blaster from Star Wars). She began shooting at me. Quick disclaimer: my son was young at the time and so my world was full of laser guns, Star Wars, force fields – you get the idea. Obviously, I didn't like being shot at, so I put a force field, like a bubble, over myself. That force field kept me from being injured. But here I was in the middle of a beautiful field, and I didn't like the idea of being confined to this force field, so I moved it to over Lynn. I took a deep breath and enjoyed the blue sky, the green grass, the lovely flowers, and the beautiful trees. Looking up, I noticed that Lynn was still firing the blaster, which was now hitting the force field, bouncing back, and wounding her. It was then that I realized that every time Lynn was shooting at me, she was also really hurting herself.

Wow, I cannot tell you how intense the wave of compassion was that hit me in that moment. On one hand it was a sad moment for me because I truly felt sad for Lynn. On the other hand, I felt huge relief because with that wave of compassion came healing to my core.

I am happy to tell you that now when I think of Lynn or see Lynn, I no longer feel a pit in my stomach. I just experience love and compassion. This was a huge transformation for me.

You see, in the moment I was able to reframe how I saw Lynn and how I saw the situation. Lynn no longer hurts me because I've decided about just how close that relationship is for me. I've set boundaries up in my life and Lynn is not in my inner circle. And now that I've looked at the situation and Lynn through a different lens, I no longer feel the intensity of hurt and pain that I used to feel.

Have you heard me excuse Lynn's behavior? Have you heard me say that what Lynn did to me was okay? Have you heard me deny that Lynn hurt me? I don't have to do any of those things to find healing. I can acknowledge the truth of the situation. I can say that her behavior in the past toward me was completely inappropriate and still find healing.

Lynn has never apologized or acknowledged her role in the situation. You see it doesn't take Lynn apologizing for me to heal. I didn't sit around waiting for her to come to me. It takes reframing on my part to find healing. And, I love myself enough to seek out that healing by doing the work that it takes to see Lynn, the situation, and myself a little differently. The work has been 100% worth it.

So, it's your turn. Do you love yourself enough to do the work that it takes to reframe Lion #1? Do it for yourself. Do it for the people who love you. Do it for your physical, spiritual, mental, and emotional well-being. Remember, you are removing a roadblock from your path to the amazing future awaiting you.

I'm proud of you! Blessings!

"Life is 10% what happens to us and 90% how we react to it."
– Dennis P. Kimbro

Day 8

Oh my goodness! Here you are reading this!!! Please know that I truly am super proud of you. This is hard work! Thank you for taking the time to invest in your life, in your future, even in your body.

Negative emotions are stored in different parts of your body. When you find emotional healing, those emotions are released from that part of your body, so your body then has the freedom to be healthier than it was before. This is the reason I got started on the journey to emotional healing. A year after my daughter was born, I was almost completely bed ridden. I had a one-year-old and a five-year-old and taking care of them was almost impossible. I was only able to do the bare minimum.

The fact that I couldn't even take care of my own children was completely unacceptable. I went from doctor to doctor trying to figure out what was wrong. I did finally find someone who could figure out all that I was dealing with in my body. It was the beginning of a holistic approach to health in my life.

We started out by addressing the physical issues. Changing my diet, rebuilding my immune system through vitamins and minerals, and taking care of things living in my body that shouldn't have been there were the building blocks to my road to healing. It didn't take long to see results from those steps. However, after time, I hit a plateau in my healing. My health had improved substantially, and I was grateful, but I wanted more.

A wise couple in my life pointed out that until I took care of the emotional side of things, the rest of the healing that I was seeking just wouldn't come. I had done tons of counseling. In fact, my mom had started me out when I was in the fifth grade.

Counseling is an amazing tool when you can find a good counselor who can walk you through the healing process. However, I felt like I had talked about my hurts until I was blue in the face. I just didn't know if that was the answer I was looking for this time around.

My journey was a process of reading, praying, talking, crying, and reading some more. It also included an amazing tool called EVOX, which is a tool by Zyto that helps to shift perceptions for a more lasting healing and change in our emotions and patterns in our lives. I learned so much during my six sessions of EVOX which catapulted me toward healing. After those sessions, I was able to see things more clearly to be able to put my tools into use. The changes I saw were enough for me to fall in love with the idea of helping others find their way and so I became an EVOX practitioner.

Addressing these negative emotions and finding healing made a HUGE impact on my physical health as well. The plateau was over. I continued to get healthier and healthier.

I want the same for you. I want physical, spiritual, mental, and emotional health for you. Dealing with the emotions locked away in parts of our bodies can also bring emotional peace as well.

Keep speaking your affirmation out loud at least twice a day. Your body, mind, and emotions will hear you and will fall in line. Be sure and tell yourself how proud you are of yourself for doing this. Keep taking the positive steps.

Today your assignment is to spend some time thinking about Lion #1. What would you do differently if you found yourself in a similar situation today? Make a list of how you would handle yourself differently. Would you speak differently? Would you act differently? Would you defend yourself? Or would you keep quiet and walk away?

Now, if you were too young to have done something differently, I want you to imagine how you, as an adult today, would help the younger version of yourself if you were present during that situation. What would that look like? What would you do? What would you say to the other people involved in Lion #1? What would you say to the younger version of yourself? Enjoy knowing that you, as an adult, would help you as a child. You can even picture rescuing yourself from that situation. You deserved the help back then and you deserve the help now.

Now, speak forgiveness over all the people involved in that situation once again. Please, please, please trust me in this. The repetition of speaking forgiveness will make a difference. I've experienced it in my own life. I've seen people experience great healing from the repetition in this process. Keep doing it. The more you do it, the deeper into your soul the forgiveness and the healing will go.

Get your assignment done and I'll meet you back here tomorrow.

Blessings!

My mission in life is not merely to survive, but to thrive; and to do so with some passion, some compassion, some humor, and some style. Maya Angelou

Day 9

I'm trusting that yesterday was helpful for you as you looked at your own actions to figure out what you would do differently if you found yourself in a similar situation. It is easy to just look at other people and see what they should do differently. It takes real courage to look at ourselves. It takes real courage to admit we would do something differently, even if that something different is standing up for ourselves.

It can be painful to look at our own actions. Regret can be powerful. You are taking steps on your path of healing! Don't give up now. Don't give in. You will be so glad you kept going.

Today is not a difficult day. Today is a day of thankfulness. You deserve a day of joy and thanksgiving!

Go back to your timeline. Speak thankfulness over each of the items above the line. Enjoy it. Be specific.

I was able to graduate from college in the midst of struggling through constant illness. I love looking back over those years and being truly thankful that I was able to persevere on the most difficult of days. I love knowing that I did that. No one else took those classes for me, no one else dragged me out of bed on days of misery and pain, no one else took all of those tests, no one else wrote all of those papers. I am so thankful that I was able to push through. I am so thankful that my parents paid for my college classes. I am so thankful for their encouragement and support. I am thankful for my friends who were there for me during difficult days. I have so much to be thankful for.

I want you to be as specific as you possibly can. Be more

specific than I have even been here. Maybe grab a cup of herbal tea and just enjoy.

I also want you to add to those things which you are thankful for. Make a list of ten things you are thankful for in your life today. Who are you thankful for? Do you have a co-worker who makes you laugh? A neighbor who smiles and waves when she sees you? A friend who never gives up on you?

What material goods are you thankful for? Do you have a roof over your head? Do you have plenty of clothes? Do you have a car? Books to read? Food in your pantry and refrigerator? What situations are you thankful for right now? A job that pays the bills? Do you have a vision for the future?

Soak it all the thankfulness and I'll see you here tomorrow.

Blessings!

"Nurture your mind with great thoughts. To believe in the heroic makes heroes." – Benjamin Disraeli

Day 10

You may be wondering what to do when Lion #1 enters your mind and brings all the negative emotions with it. You know how it is.... You're just sitting there minding your own business when the situation pops into your mind and you find yourself reliving that situation over again. I don't know about you, but this happens most frequently when I have some downtime or I'm lying in bed at night. The sadness, anger, frustration, and the other negative emotions can then settle in and get much too comfortable.

This is where some discipline (and some trust in me) comes into play. Each time that Lion #1 pops into your mind, I want you to stop these thoughts immediately. How do you do that? You are going to stop whatever you are doing and say, out loud, "No! I've already forgiven _____ (fill in the blank with the name of the person involved). I choose healing. I choose joy and peace."

Practice this. Say it forcefully. Let your mind know that this thought process is completely unacceptable. After you've done it multiple times, it will start to become second nature. Keep doing it, every single time. This takes practice and repetition. Sometimes you will catch yourself at the very beginning of thoughts of Lion #1. Sometimes you will have allowed your mind to go down that pit before you stop yourself. The more you do it, the earlier you will catch yourself.

After you have stopped the repetitive thoughts of Lion #1, you will need to fill your mind with other thoughts. Go into speaking thankfulness or find a fun, positive song to sing. Memorize an inspirational quote to repeat. Or, go into speaking an affirmation. You've stopped the thoughts now fill your mind with something uplifting and encouraging.

I know that some of you are feeling very skeptical at this point. Please, for your emotional health, trust me on this one. After five times of doing this you will be well on your way to developing a habit and you will feel a difference. Your mind and body will obey your will. You've already done so much work in this area, so now it is time to stop the madness in its tracks. Do not let Lion #1 steal one more minute from your life! Take control of it now.

The more you practice saying, "No!…." when Lion #1 rears its ugly head, the more you will feel the forgiveness. The more you practice, the smaller a hold that Lion #1 will have over you. The more you practice, the more freedom you will experience.

Your assignment isn't just about today. Your assignment is about every day for the rest of your life. You won't have to keep taking those thoughts captive for the rest of your life, they will eventually just fade; however, new life situations will come and this will be a tool to put in your belt to pull out when needed.

Trust me, this is a powerful tool! I love watching the hurt and pain fade in my life. I love feeling deep forgiveness for others. I love getting to let go of regret. It took me a long time to learn this mostly because I didn't actually believe that it would work so I didn't practice it. I hope you learn quickly, practice often, and enjoy the fruits of your labor.

Blessings!

"Courage is the first of human qualities because it is the quality which guarantees all others." – Winston Churchill

Day 11

Hello, friend! Again, let me tell you how wonderfully proud I am of you, your hard work, your perseverance, and your love for yourself. Keep moving forward and let's see where you end up.

Today you are going to take out your timeline and write "forgiven and healed" over Lion #1. You are going to need to trust me on this one. Do it, even if you don't feel healed. Do it, even if you don't feel the peace that comes with complete and total forgiveness and healing. Your body, mind, and emotions will fall in line. They will follow the decisions that you make. It is amazing to watch and experience the changes that come with making these decisions, following through with them, and repeating them. You are creating new pathways in your brain, new patterns of dealing with life challenges, and new tools for anything you might encounter in life.

I also want you to make another list of ten things you are thankful for. Be sure to add being thankful for the healing you are experiencing with Lion #1 (even if you don't feel it). Remember all of this is what you have chosen. I didn't used to believe that all of this was a choice, mostly because I didn't experience immediate relief. What I've figured out is that it requires repetition. So, repeat the thankfulness and the forgiveness!!!

I'm looking forward to seeing you tomorrow!!!

"The great thing in this world is not so much where you stand, as in what direction you are moving." – Oliver Wendell Holmes

Day 12

Today we'll begin working on the second Lion of the three most negatively impactful. Now, it may seem to you that we are going through these quickly and you'd be right. We don't want to spend the next ten years healing from events that have already stolen so much from you.

Don't get me wrong, there are often layers to healing. So, if we can work on the first layer and find healing there, then the next layer may take care of itself. At the very least, you'll find the next layer easier to address or you'll feel more confident about addressing it.

I've found that as I start addressing the layers, then the event doesn't affect me as strongly or as deeply. And, sometimes I'll be hit with something that in the past would have been a trigger for emotional turmoil; however, I'm surprised to find that the past work I've done for my emotional well-being has allowed me to move on to the point where I'm no longer bothered. You see, as you work through these things and demand that your mind and emotions follow the will, you find that other healing has taken place. Something that would have been a trigger in the past won't bother you like before. The work will be worth it!

Okay, so let's dig in. Take Lion #2 and make a list of all the people involved. Let's make sure that you include yourself in this list.

"Either you run the day, or the day runs you." – Jim Rohn

Day 13

Okay, so you already know the drill. Today you are going to go through your list of people involved in Lion #2. Speak forgiveness over each person on your list, including yourself. Do this out loud. I like to say it emphatically to make sure that my mind knows that I'm completely serious and committed to the idea of forgiving this person. And, yes, I say it even if I'm not *feeling* it. You are in charge of your emotions, not the other way around.

This is another big decision day for you. Are you going to keep drinking the poison that you have made for someone else? Are you going to allow that person, that situation to be an obstacle on your journey in life? Do you really want that person to be the reason you don't achieve all that you could, to be the reason you don't have the relationships you want, to be the reason you are miserable?

You are here, so I know the answer to those questions. You are ready to find freedom from the pain, the hurt, the unforgiveness. This is one of the best decisions you will ever make. You'll look back and be proud of yourself. You'll be so thrilled with the results!

"_____ (insert that person's name), when you _____ (fill in their part in Lion #2), that really hurt my feelings (or put in what you felt at that time, anger, frustration, sadness, etc.). Today I choose to forgive you, _____ (insert their name) for your part in _____ (Lion #2). I choose to let go of that hurt today. I choose joy and peace right now because I deserve joy and peace."

Remember, if you were too young to have done anything about this situation, then what I want you to do is speak something like this toward yourself:

"_____ (insert your name), when _____ (Lion #2) happened you were not at fault. You were a child, and the adults were responsible for taking care of you. This was not your fault. I love you. I do not hold you responsible for what happened."

You love yourself enough to choose life, joy, healing, and peace! Awesomeness!!!

Please remember to keep saying your affirmation multiple times a day.

"The difference between a successful person and others is not lack of strength not a lack of knowledge but rather a lack of will." – Vince Lombardi

Day 14

It's reframing day! Start by taking out your timeline and write "forgiven and healed" over Lion #2. This is about taking charge of your emotions. Let your will dictate what will happen in your life.

Today is not about excuses. There will be no denial. We are just going to take Lion #2 and start looking at it from different angles. I want you to see the whys behind the behaviors of the people involved.

What negative events have these people been through in their past that might have predisposed them to behave this way?

What was going on in their lives when Lion #2 occurred?

What are some hurts they are still carrying?

Again, please don't hear me excusing their behavior! We all have to take responsibility for our actions. However, when we can feel what someone else might be feeling it helps us to understand the whys behind their actions. This makes the forgiveness process a little easier, a little less painful.

The other person may or may not ever know that you experienced empathy for them and their situation, but you will know. The anger, hurt, and frustration will dissipate. Isn't that what we are after? Healing, peace, and greater joy?

As you begin to see the reasons behind others' hurtful behaviors, speak forgiveness toward those people. Yes, I know you've spoken forgiveness toward these people, but say it again. I know this process works, so keep doing the work.

Be sure and look at yourself too. Do not excuse or deny your own behaviors, but instead try to understand the whys behind your behaviors. Forgive yourself. Speak it out loud. Give yourself lots of grace. Let go of any regret you feel about Lion #2. Show yourself the same compassion and kindness that you would show to your closest friend. You need to be your own friend too!

"It always seems impossible until it's done." Nelson Mandela

Day 15

Are you saying your affirmations at least twice a day? This is truly important. Think of it as rewiring your brain. This takes time and effort. Think of your thoughts as traveling down roads inside your mind. Your thoughts are used to traveling the same old roads, even comfortable traveling the same old roads. BUT, as you begin to choose different roads, your mind will automatically start choosing those new roads. You don't need the old roads any longer. They are not helping you; they're hindering you. Maybe you needed those old roads for a period of time, but today is the day to build new roads, new ways of thinking. Let's keep choosing the new roads that lead to a happier, healthier you!

Now for today's assignment! Today you are going to examine Lion #2 and ask yourself what you would do differently if you found yourself in the same situation today. You can't change anyone else's behavior, but you can change your own. You can look forward to the future and prepare yourself for similar situations that might come your way.

Let's say your boss is having a really bad day at work. Oh, by the way, what you don't know is that your boss's child was diagnosed with an incurable disease two days ago. Anyway, back to the bad day at work. You don't particularly like how he's talking to you, so you get angry and yell at him. Later that day human resources calls you in for a little talk. You had another incident a few months ago, so this is your second incident on your record. Human resource decides that is enough to let you go. You lose your job.

Maybe your boss was being a total jerk and what he was saying to you was completely out of line. However, it wasn't his behavior that got you fired. It was your behavior.

You see, you are going to come across more jerks, or more people who are hurting deeply, in the future. You must decide how you are going to handle your own behavior when you do come across them.

So, now you get to look at that situation with new eyes. How would you handle that situation differently in the future? Let's do that with Lion #2. Please remember that our goal is healing and growth. You may not enjoy this process, but you are investing in your future. Denial will not serve you well. Facing the truth, facing your mistakes, facing shortfalls, and facing regrets is important. You are worth it!

Remember, if you were too young to have protected yourself or stood up for yourself, I want you to imagine how you, as an adult today, would help the younger version of yourself if you were present during that situation. What would that look like? What would you do? What would you say to the other people involved in Lion #2? What would you say to the younger version of yourself? Enjoy knowing that you, as an adult, would help you as a child. You can even picture rescuing yourself from that situation. You deserved the help back then and you deserve the help now. So, step in and help the younger version of yourself.

When you get done, be sure and speak forgiveness over each person involved, especially yourself. Remember we are constructing new roads. We are leaving behind old behaviors, old ways of thinking, old paths.

I'll say it again and again that you are worth it!

The most difficult thing is the decision to act, the rest is merely tenacity. –Amelia Earhart

Day 16

Today I want you to go back to your above the line list. Again, speak thankfulness over each item you listed. You see, our brains can get in a rut of thinking about only the negative. It can become our constant focus – I know, I used to be there. Our culture is also a negative culture. You have to fight for the positive. You have to fight for thankfulness. You have to choose to focus on the good.

As you go about your days, ask yourself if what you are spending your time and energy on is helping you or hurting you. Stop and think about what you are watching on TV. Are the shows that you are watching positive and encouraging? Or, are they dark, negative, and taking your mind places you don't really want it to go, that aren't really good for you? What about the movies you are going to see? Are they helping you to pave new roads in your mind or are they getting in the way of construction?

Have you paid attention to the lyrics of most music? I don't care what genre of music you enjoy, if it has lyrics, most of it is incredibly negative. It is so funny how picky I've become about my music. I used to like the sad and depressing lyrics because it allowed me to wallow in my own misery. Since I'm no longer wallowing, I just refuse to listen to that stuff. I deserve better! So, frequently I'll hear the beginning of a song I used to love, and I'll get all excited about it. Oh, then they start singing and I start thinking. Then, I change the station. I'm not going to let all of my hard work go to waste on some song that I used to love. I love myself way more than I love some negative, depressing song.

I might step on some toes here and I know, because I used to be a news junky. I'm not saying that you should stop watching the news. Obviously, we should all be informed on what is going on in the world around us. But here's the deal, the media makes money being dramatic and repeating that drama over and over and over again. You could seriously watch about ten minutes or spend ten minutes reading the highlights of the day's news online and then move on. There are very few people in this world who need to sit and watch the news for hours on end. I used to get caught up in the news of the day, allowing it to affect my mind and emotions. What a waste all of that was for me.

Same ideas go for social media. Facebook, Twitter, Instagram, and all of the others can be great ways for us to connect with friends, family, and colleagues; however, we've all gotten worked up over some horrible post. We should all practice reading a post and then just moving on without allowing it to control our emotions. Or, unless you are using it for your livelihood, maybe we should all spend a little less time seeing what the rest of the world is up to. Wouldn't it be better for us to spend our time learning, growing, breathing, and taking care of ourselves and those we love?

What I'm asking you to do is to think, think, think. We are all used to just cruising through life. Let's shift into a different gear. Vegging out is fun and useful sometimes, but engaging our brains is necessary for a blessed life. So, please think about what you are reading, watching, and listening to. Choose only the best for yourself and watch the positive effects roll in!

Twenty years from now you will be more disappointed by the things that you didn't do than by the ones you did do, so throw off the bowlines, sail away from safe harbor, catch the trade winds in your sails. Explore, Dream, Discover. –Mark Twain

Day 17

Okay, my friend, let's tackle Lion #3. Once again you are going to make a list of all the people involved including yourself. Keep trusting me on this.

I hope you are excited about the positive results that you KNOW are coming with the work you are going to do with Lion #3. There is more sunshine coming in your life. There is more joy. There is more Life! How do I know that? The answer is that I've done this myself. I've done this work. My life is happier, more joyful, more peaceful. You cannot imagine how badly I want that for you too. I can imagine you're sitting and reading this book, dealing with sadness, depression, and deep pain, and then moving through these exercises. Now I'm imagining your experiencing forgiveness for others and for yourself. You are feeling lighter, less burdened, less angry, more relaxed, happier. That is exciting!!!! That brings me great joy!

I know that some of this has been hard. I know that there have been tears shed, anger felt. You've faced emotions that were challenging to face, but you are worth it! Please hear me! In fact, I want you to say it out loud. Say, "I am worth it!" Keep saying it until you believe it. Thank you for investing in your future and thank you for hanging in there with me.

The best time to plant a tree was 20 years ago. The second-best time is now. –Chinese Proverb

Day 18

Off we go with Lion #3. Speak forgiveness toward each of the people involved. Remember that this is an act of the will. Your emotions will follow. Just keep at it.

"_____ (insert that person's name), when you _____ (fill in their part in Lion #3), that really hurt my feelings (or put in what you felt at that time, anger, frustration, sadness, etc.). Today I choose to forgive you, _____ (insert their name) for your part in _____ (Lion #3). I choose to let go of that hurt today. I choose joy and peace right now because I deserve joy and peace."

Remember that if you were a child and unable to have done anything about this situation, then speak something like this toward yourself:

"_____ (insert your name), when _____ (Lion #3) happened you were not at fault. You were a child and the adults were responsible for taking care of you. This was not your fault. I love you. I do not hold you responsible for what happened."

Remember when the situation comes up in your mind in the future and you begin to feel the negative emotions, just stop what you are doing and say, "NO! I've already forgiven them for that. I choose freedom and joy." Be in control over your emotions. Do not let them control you. Be in charge!

I am extremely proud of you. I hope you are proud of yourself!

An unexamined life is not worth living. –Socrates

Day 19

Let's look at Lion #3 through a different lens today. Start by taking time and writing "forgiven and healed" over Lion #3.

Now, let's think about the people involved and try to see deeper into what was going on with each of them. Can we find some compassion for them? No excusing their bad or inappropriate behavior, but we need to just see people for the mess that they are. We all have our issues. If we can look into the hearts and minds of those people that have hurt us, we can gain a deeper understanding. Maybe they are in desperate need of freedom, the kind of freedom that you are pursuing through this process.

"It does not matter how slowly you go as long as you do not stop." Confucius

Let's do it. I'm behind you. I'm cheering for you!

Day 20

Think about how far you've come in the previous 19 days. You may be feeling great or you may be feeling down and discouraged. They are both normal. If you are feeling discouraged, know that you could be going through a detox of sorts. When we are facing and letting go of negative emotions, we really can experience mental, physical, and emotional symptoms. Know that they will go away. Be sure that you are drinking lots of water. Remember, drinking half your weight in ounces is a good rule of thumb. So, if you weigh 200 pounds, you will want to be drinking around 100 ounces of water each day. Coffee, tea, sodas, and juice do not count. It needs to be pure water.

I also want to make sure that you are eating healthy. Your body needs to be supported while you are doing this work. It is just as easy to stop at a healthy grocery store and buy a healthy meal as it is to stop at fast food after a long day at work. And, your body will feel better the next day.

Exercise is also such a great support during this time. Please don't think that is has to be some incredibly intense bodybuilding workout. Nothing wrong with those, but keep in mind that even a walk around the block can make a huge impact on your body, mind, and emotions. When I'm upset, I find that a walk in my neighborhood helps to burn off negative emotions. I feel relief with each step I take. There are so many great workout videos online that are free if you need something to do inside on a day with bad weather.

And don't forget the benefits of sunshine. Sunshine is what our bodies need to produce vitamin D. Vitamin D is great for our moods. And doesn't the sun on your skin just feel wonderful?

This is all about taking care of yourself, inside and out! Keep pushing through, keep saying your affirmation, and know that any discouragement that comes will pass.

Today I want you to look back on Lion #3 and assess your own part in the situation. What could you have done differently? This truly takes a lot of courage and maturity on your part. AND, it moves you closer to your healing! YES!!!

Again, if you were a child at the time and couldn't have done anything differently, then ask yourself what you would do as an adult in the same situation. What would you say? What would you do? What would you say to your younger self? What would you do for your younger self?

As you practice this exercise, it will get easier. You'll learn and grow. You'll get more proficient. It's like when someone is learning how to read. They take one step at a time, learning the letters, then learning the sounds the letters make, then blending the letters together and then forming words. It takes time, effort, energy, and practice. These exercises also take practice. If you find that you are discouraged, take a deep breath, get a good night of sleep, and then start again tomorrow.

You can never cross the ocean until you have the courage to lose sight of the shore. –Christopher Columbus

Day 21

Today you are going to make a new list of all the things you can be thankful for. Why a new list? Because your perspective has changed over the past three weeks. You are beginning to see through new eyes. You'll continue to feel gratitude on a deeper level the further you go on this journey. This will also become a daily habit for you. You'll find new things to be thankful for.

Quite possibly you need the encouragement from a thankfulness list. Maybe you need to pause and feel the impact of the things around you that make you happy. Pause, breathe, and enjoy your list.

Keep choosing joy, healing, and peace! You are so worth it. Enjoy the thankfulness. Smile!

People often say that motivation doesn't last. Well, neither does bathing. That's why we recommend it daily. –Zig Ziglar

Day 22

Oh, today is one of my favorite days! It's REWARD DAY! When I think about all of the hard work you have put into this process, I just want to take you out for dinner or go hiking with you. You deserve a reward for everything you've persevered through over the past three weeks.

Since I can't take you out for dinner and chat with you, I want you to find a way to reward yourself. That reward could be a nice long walk, a dinner with a friend, a fun conversation with your spouse over a cup of herbal tea, or a fun gift for yourself. You get to decide what feels like a reward to you. What I get excited about might not be what you get excited about.

If you can't make that reward happen today, I want you to be sure and get it on your calendar. Text a friend and pick a night to have dinner. Please hear me be emphatic about this! You need to get this nailed down. Some of you will get excited and I don't have to push you to make this happen, but others won't see the importance of this. Trust me, this is important. When you are sipping that cup of tea while watching the sunset, you'll be thinking about how proud you are of yourself for all of your hard work. Your body, mind and emotions will take notice and will want to do whatever it takes to make that happen again.

You need to make sure that this reward is truly a reward. Just because we enjoy something doesn't mean it is good for us. Going out to dinner is wonderful, but if we overeat and then the next day feel badly about ourselves because we overate or if it was too much for our digestive system, then we didn't really reward ourselves, we actually punished ourselves. If we go out and partake of anything that makes us feel badly later, then we are not rewarding ourselves.

Make sure it is a positive reward, something that will make you smile, laugh, and feel good about yourself. Go for a walk in a park you've never been to before, schedule a massage, buy that new pair of shoes you've been needing, pick up that book you've been wanting to read, plan a campout, or take a long bath while listening to some relaxing music.

I have a tea place that I absolutely love, Dubs Tea and Water. One of my favorite things is to stop in and pick up some unsweet, cinnamon roll iced tea. It makes me smile and I never regret drinking some. That is truly a reward for me. I also love getting to have dinner with my husband or with a friend. Oh, and a nice long hike in nature makes me happy too. All of those make me happy. Getting dinner out with my husband or with a friend often requires looking ahead and putting the date on my calendar. However, stopping by my favorite tea spot can be a spontaneous reward.

So, take a few minutes to think what you want your reward to be and plan it or do it. Another fun option would be to plan a fun getaway. However, if you choose this option, make sure that it is on the calendar within the next 28 days. You don't want to reward yourself a year from now, you want to reward yourself now. Don't put it off. Oh, and feel free to do multiple rewards. You've done so much work, you deserve it! Just take good care of yourself.

Go confidently in the direction of your dreams. Live the life you have imagined. –Henry David Thoreau

Day 23

Okay, I'm really hoping that yesterday you did a great job of rewarding yourself or getting the reward on the calendar! Please know that you have done so much hard work and you truly do deserve some fun! This is part of taking care of yourself, so make it happen! If you didn't do it yesterday, then make it happen today.

Today your assignment is to make a list of the six most influential people in your life. These can be parents, siblings, spouses, children, best friends, teachers, spiritual leaders, coworkers, or mentors. Now spend a little time speaking thankfulness for each of these people, for the help they've been in your life, for what they mean to you, and for what you've learned from them. You don't have to actually do this in front of the person, just do it out loud in the privacy of your own home.

I love really thinking through the people in my life who have made a huge impact in my life. Some are no longer here with us and I miss them terribly, but I love getting to reminisce. Thinking back on lessons taught, the hugs given, and the encouragement poured out just makes me smile.

Enjoy!

Do what you can, where you are, with what you have. –Teddy Roosevelt

Day 24

Today you are going to pick two of the six most influential people in your life that you listed yesterday. I want you to imagine one of those people sitting across from you. Tell that person what you appreciate about them. Do this *out loud*. Really think through this. What do you want them to know? What is on your mind and in your heart?

Now I want you to tell them things you wish they had done differently. Don't gloss over this just because you love, admire, or appreciate this person. Really think. What do you need them to know that may have hurt your feelings? What did they not do that you wish they had done? It's okay to tell them that you wish they had done something a little differently. They aren't sitting across from you, so you can't hurt their feelings. However, this could be a great opportunity for you to get some negative emotions out of your body. And, you know the drill. Be sure and speak forgiveness toward them for the things that may have hurt your feelings or just left you feeling some sort of loss.

You're getting really good at speaking forgiveness! You're going to just love how it makes you feel. FREEDOM! If you aren't feeling it yet, just keep practicing. You'll get there, I promise!

Repeat this exercise with influential person #2. Remember appreciation, releasing negative emotions, and speaking forgiveness. And be sure you are doing all of this *out loud*.

Are you still saying your affirmation? Be a blessing to yourself by continuing in that habit.

If the wind will not serve, take to the oars. –Latin Proverb

Day 25

Today you are going to repeat the same thing you did yesterday with two more people. What do you love and appreciate about these two people and what do you wish they had done differently? Speak forgiveness.

Have you noticed that you are on Day 25? Pure awesomeness! I am beyond proud of all of your hard work. You've removed barriers to your future, forgiven multiple people, forgiven yourself, spoken your affirmation daily, and practiced thankfulness. All of this is so huge!!! You truly will experience more joy, freedom, grace, and love in your life because of this work. We all want more of those in our lives, but not everyone will put in the time and effort to get there.

I have learned over the years that when one's mind is made up, this diminishes fear. –Rosa Parks

Day 26

Welcome back! Here we are at the home stretch! Keep pushing through until the end. Each and every day that you keep going is another day closer to your goals. I truly wish I could hug you to congratulate you!

Today you are going to speak to the last two of the six most influential people in your life. Appreciation is important because it reminds us that we have had people in our lives who have been of support and encouragement. I had an English teacher, Mrs. Peters, in the seventh grade who always smiled at me when she saw me in the hall and when I walked into her classroom. Even that simple act made my year so much better. Maybe that doesn't seem like a big impact, but it was to me during that challenging year in my life. So, I've spoken appreciation toward Mrs. Peters, and it was really fun to do.

What are you experiencing when you speak that appreciation? Sit in it for a few minutes and really enjoy that feeling. Enjoy the memories.

Remember to tell these two people what you wish they had done differently, even if they are small things. And, then forgiveness must follow that. Release those negative emotions. Set yourself free.

The question isn't who is going to let me; it's who is going to stop me. –Ayn Rand

Day 27

Today I want you to picture those six influential people sitting in the room with you. Speak forgiveness again over each and every one of those people. I know, I know you've been doing this over the past few days. Please trust me. The repetition is powerful! You don't have to relive what they did, you are just speaking forgiveness and choosing a more beautiful and fulfilling life.

Forgiveness is an act of the will, and the will can function regardless of the temperature of the heart. — Corrie Ten Boom

Day 28

CONGRATULATIONS!!!! Oh my goodness! Here you are at Day 28! You've invested in your life! Know that your determination to get to Day 28 shows your love for yourself. And it's much easier to love other people if you love yourself first. Not only will your life be better, but your relationships will be better, so the lives of the people you love will be better too. Success in life, work, and relationships will come so much more easily because of the work you have done and will continue to do. What a gift!

As you move forward you will have two assignments that will carry you through life.

1. Keep speaking your affirmation out loud. Write new ones as you grow and change. Keep incorporating them into your life. You are using these to re-wire your brain for success, joy, peace, love, and life.

2. When those old Lions come up in your mind, you now know how to handle them. You are going to say, out loud, "No! I've already forgiven _____. I choose joy and peace and love!" Then speak your affirmation out loud. You see, you get to decide whether those Lions stay Lions or become Flies. Keep choosing for those Lions to be downgraded. The more you stop the thoughts from taking over, the easier it will become to make those thoughts submit. The pain and hurts no longer get to run your life. Keep taking your life back any time those negative thoughts show up and threaten to take over.

Don't judge each day by the harvest you reap but by the seeds that you plant. --Robert Louis Stevenson

74

Part III

Now What?

I know some of you are not feeling deep healing and relief. Know that that is okay. It took me a while to push through all the blockades that I faced in this process. I still have some lions (that are becoming flies) that will rear their ugly heads and I have to speak forgiveness over that situation again. But here's the deal, I don't have to do it very often any longer and it has become much easier, with practice, to put those issues to rest.

You have to love yourself and be strong enough to persevere. Some days this was difficult for me and some days it was easy. Some days I did not accomplish what I set out to accomplish. Some days I fell into depression and self-loathing. When I didn't capture the ugliness, I found myself held captive to the hurts and pains. However, when I made the decision to pursue forgiveness and my own peaceful future, I found that each day brought further joy, peace, and deeper self-love.

So, keep practicing forgiveness with the lions you've already worked on. And, now you have other lions to work on. Do this because you know it is going to bring relief. Do this because you love yourself. Do this because you'll find freedom.

Take this one day at a time. Just don't give up on yourself. Repetition is the key. Our brains, our emotions are wonderfully made. They are resilient and have the wonderful ability to change and grow. However, it does take work. You do have to fight for this. Some of the lions you have left on your list will heal quickly. Others will take more time. And some will feel completely healed and yet one day you'll get hit with an emotion that surprises you. Just think of this as peeling another layer in the onion of healing on that particular lion. You are working toward deeper healing as you face each layer.

Be sure and write forgiven over each of your lions. It's just a reminder that you have worked through that particular issue. And then keep speaking forgiveness over each of the layers of those issues as you come across them.

I have to tell you that I have experienced so much hope through this process, because I know that as new things arise healing can be found in those too. I don't get so bogged down in discouragement any longer, because I know with taking these lions captive I'll find healing. Lions used to make me feel hopeless because I didn't know how to achieve healing. The past work lets me know that healing is just around the corner. This is true for you too.

Will I really find permanent healing?

Jonathan (his name has been changed) is a man who came to see me seeking healing. He's in his late forties and in a lot of deep pain. He came to see me three times and all of our sessions were exactly the same. I'd listen to him tell part of his story and I'd give him assignments. I truly felt very sorry for Jonathan. He dealt with so much shame, embarrassment, and loneliness. The hurt that he had from some really dumb, hurtful things his parents had said and done was etched all over his face. His voice was weak and it sounded like it was physically painful for him to talk. I showed him compassion and reassured him that he had suffered an injustice.

I knew, from experience, after our first session together that he wouldn't find healing unless he changed his mentality. I even told him this. You see, Jonathan was convinced that he had done all of the work and that nothing changed his pain. He didn't believe that the work we did would change anything. I wondered if he somehow really liked being the sad case that he was. I don't say that to be mean, I say that to remind us of all that we have to be willing to let go of pain and accept healing. He just wouldn't let go.

I still think about Jonathan. I hope he's okay and that at some point he made a decision to truly pursue his own healing.

You see Jonathan had said affirmations, lots of them. The difference is that Jonathan believed, at one point, that just saying them over and over would change his emotions and circumstances. What Jonathan didn't understand and wasn't open to learning was that he needed to choose to believe the affirmations. He also wouldn't stop the ugly thoughts that came in his head. He would entertain the hurt and pain for hours at a time. He'd been entertaining the demons in his head for years and he just kept on entertaining them.

Jonathan wouldn't listen to me. He didn't want to be told to stop the madness. He was stuck replaying the same bad movie over and over again. He needed to push stop. Each time the movie started to play again, he needed to push stop. He wasn't willing to push stop. Maybe he felt entitled to hold on to the pain and hurt. Unfortunately, Jonathan is his own worst enemy. He couldn't hear that he was hurting himself day in and day out. He wouldn't forgive. He wouldn't choose to stop the madness that screamed at him in his head. He wouldn't take control. Now, I'm not being hard on Jonathan. I only say these things because I've been there. I know what it feels like to let the madness run wild. My life changed when I made the decision to stop the crazy thoughts in my head and speak forgiveness toward myself and others.

New patterns had to be made in my life and new patterns need to be made in Jonathan's life. You've started on this journey making new patterns in your life. Do not give up on yourself. Making these new patterns takes time and work. If you will persevere and do the work, then yes, deep, permanent healing will take place in your life. How do I know? Because I've experienced it myself and have helped hundreds of people do the same.

Toxic Relationships

If you are in an abusive relationship, please get help. Do not stay in that relationship expecting the other person to change. You can only change you. Abusers usually make sure the person they are abusing feels at fault. This is their way of controlling the situation and the person they are abusing. It keeps the abuser from feeling guilt and shame as well. Stop believing that it is your fault that person is hitting you, sexually abusing you, playing horrible mental games with you, screaming at you, threatening you, and calling you horrible names. They will say that things didn't really happen the way you say they happened. They will make you second guess yourself. Please, get help. My favorite resource for help in this area is Leslie Vernick. You can find her at www.leslievernick.com

There are also relationships that just don't fit with our new outlook on life. I'm not saying throw away your relationships! Don't make the mistake of getting rid of everyone while you are super excited about your new path. You never know, those people may join you. You could be the one to lead them in a new positive direction.

If you find yourself having conversations with friends who are negative or talk negatively about others, try to change the subject. Don't force it or try to make them feel badly about being negative, just steer the conversation in a different direction. Be careful doing this. You don't want to come across as judgmental or that you are feeling superior. However, you also don't want to continue down that path. Being negative and gossiping about others is not what you are about any longer. Eleanor Roosevelt once said, "Great minds discuss ideas; average minds discuss events; small minds discuss people." Focus on ideas when spending time with friends and family. If they cannot join you in discussing ideas, then focus on events.

This may not go over very well. Your friends and family members may not appreciate the change in the relationship. They may want you to stay as you were, negative, angry, hurting. You'll need to make the decision to stay the course in spite of the frustration of others. And, you don't have to kick them out of your life. Trust me, people who don't like the changes you've made will excuse themselves out of your life on their own.

You may also find yourself changing your activities. Where before you engaged in unproductive activities, you are now making healthier choices. This again may cull people out of your life. This may be painful, my friend, but know that surrounding yourself with people who love you and want the very best for you will be so worth it in the long run. There may be a bit of loneliness as you transition from unhealthy relationships to healthier ones, but one day you'll look up and find yourself with new friends who truly support you.

How and where do I find these new people? I believe that changing your attitude will naturally draw people to you. You'll have conversations at work that are positive with people you've never really interacted with, and those conversations will turn into more conversations. If you've decided to change your physical health along with these new emotional changes, then find others who are interested in healthier physical choices. A gym, healthy cooking classes, or a neighborhood walking group are good choices. If you can't find exactly what you are looking for, then start a group yourself. People who are working to be healthy attract others who are working toward better health. Start a book club and choose positive, life-changing books. Start a new hobby and you'll find others who are passionate about that hobby. As you think and talk about ideas, find others out there who want to talk about ideas as well. Find a business club or a study group that is focused on personal growth. Positive, healthy people are out there, just keep making healthy choices and those friendships will come.

Okay, but what about family? This one is a little tricky. We can choose our friends (people who often become like family), but we can't choose those we are related to. Really, I see this coming down to two options. You can choose to pull away a little bit and just not spend as much time with family who are bringing you down or you can choose to direct these relationships in a more positive direction.

Again, please be careful when you pull away. There is no need to announce the pulling away because that will only cause hurt. You aren't looking to cause pain to your family members. Maybe just choose to have fewer phone conversations or when you answer the phone let them know that you only have a set amount of time to talk because you have something you need to take care of. You can also choose to gather with family less frequently. Love them enough to give them a chance to change too. Remember, you have grown and changed and so can they.

What would it look like to direct these relationships in a more positive direction? Try to meet them where they are. Do they love to read? Recommend reading a book together to talk about it. You choose the book, of course. Do they love movies? Find positive, up-lifting, inspiring movies that you can watch together. Go on walks together. Choose fun, outdoor activities. You can also think ahead of time topics of conversation that are more positive and encouraging. Ask questions about that person that would lead toward mutual encouragement. This will help steer the conversation in a direction that benefits you both. All of this will require prep work.

Really, you can use the same strategies for all your

relationships. Be the guiding force. Plan in advance. This is not insincere. In fact, this shows how much you really care about your relationships. Taking the time to invest in the relationships is the most sincere, kind, and loving way to bless those around you.

Building Healthy Relationships with Friends and Family

Isolation from friends and family can also be toxic. And I think sometimes when our perception is off, we forget how to connect with others. So, let's find some ways to cultivate deeper, more fulfilling relationships, shall we?

Researchers say that people that eat together have closer relationships. Sitting around with mouths full of food isn't what brings the people closer. Conversations, questions, and active listening make for beautiful times of intimacy among friends and family.

Most of us have strong memories of some mealtimes with family. Those may be good memories or bad memories. They could be daily mealtimes or only special occasions. If your early memories are not pleasant, then go ahead and admit it and then make the determination that what goes into your meals times with family and friends will be different than your childhood memories. And, if this is your case, then you might even be more creative than someone who has good memories. You have no preconceived ideas. Embrace the freedom to make this your own. If your mealtime memories are lovely, then be excited about recreating those memories.

So, let's get down to the practical ways to have fun and interesting mealtimes to build memories. You can start with something as simple as highs and lows of the day. What was your favorite part of the day and what was the worst thing that happened today? Those two answers will give great insight into how everyone's day went. You'll also have a jumping off point for further conversation. Usually, the answers to those questions will prompt you to ask deeper questions. Also, keep in mind that we all love to be asked questions about ourselves. The person who is being asked will walk away from mealtime feeling loved and valued. Trust is built in this exercise and can help everyone to be authentic with each other and others. If honest and transparent sharing is occurring, then make sure it is a safe place. Obviously be careful how deeply you share with certain people and always make sure that you guard closely the information that others share with you. This is a great way to develop allies in life.

Mealtime is also a great time to talk about your plans for a new healthy life and an exciting future. Sharing your plans will also give you some accountability to keep moving forward. Ask your friends and family members about their hopes and dreams too. You can then be of support for one another.

If there is a person talking, then obviously there will also be people listening. Eye contact lets a person know that you are listening, caring, and sharing in what they are saying. But you can also take this one step further. Active listening is when you paraphrase back to someone what they said. This reassures the person that you've heard what they've said, but also that you understand what they are trying to communicate. We all like to be heard and understood. Active listening can make someone feel very special and loved.

I have several friends who are verbal processors. These are people who need to talk to sort out what is going on inside their heads. When those friends talk, I can bet that most of the time it is to organize thoughts and provide solutions to their own problems. When we listen to that person, we can see the stress melting off their shoulders. Usually this only takes a few minutes of our time and the investment is more than worth it. If you are a verbal processor, find friends who are willing to let you process through all that is rolling around in your head. However, always make sure you balance the talking with listening.

Getting friends and family out of the house, away from distractions (assuming you don't bring the distractions with you) provides communication, fresh air, memory building, bonding, and exercise. So, let's get back to the distractions. Facebook, email, Pinterest, texts, and other forms of media are constantly surrounding us and bombarding us. These keep us from connecting with the people that we love. On your walks, leave your phones and all other devices at home. It will be okay for you to be unreachable for thirty minutes. The world will not come to an end. This will give you the ability to focus on the people who are present in the moment which gives you more time to love on one another, get to know one another, and enjoy each other.

Electronics are often brain-numbing. Pulling our brains out of all of that will be refreshing for you and your friends as well. I find that we all seem to have better moods when we have spent time outdoors exercising. Good attitudes can be contagious.

This is another great time to ask thought-provoking questions. A question that will either get to the heart or will prompt deep thought and discussion is: What are you passionate about? Another way to reconnect is to make a game of it. Guess how you think a person will answer questions such as: What is your favorite movie? What is your favorite color? What is your favorite book? What is your favorite activity? Have fun and laugh!

Your walks can also be a great educational activity. Buy a book or a field guide about trees, flowers, birds, or butterflies. Learn how to identify different species together. Once you get good at spotting the different types, you can make a game of it. How many different types of trees can you identify in your neighborhood? Find out what your family and friends might be interested in studying.

There is something to be said for getting out of our houses and getting a little exercise. Going on a walk can produce endorphins which makes us happier. We all want happier friends and family members, right? Exercise also makes us healthier. A twenty-minute walk is so good for our bodies. It is simple, doesn't take a lot of equipment or time; however, memories are being built that will last a lifetime.

There are endless possibilities to hobbies that you can choose to participate in with those you love. Make sure that the hobby you choose is something that everyone will enjoy doing together. We all have different personalities and have different interests. This needs to be an all-inclusive interest.

You can even spend some time brainstorming, with your friends, ideas for hobbies that you might enjoy together. If you are thinking about outdoor hobbies, then gardening might be a good choice. In our microwave-paced life, gardening can provide great perspective. There are seasons to gardening, there is time, waiting and patience involved, and a connection to the reality of life. There is something wonderfully satisfying to planting seeds, watering those seeds, seeing the first plants emerge from the ground, protecting the plants from harsh weather, drought or insects, harvesting what has been nurtured and then eating the fruits of labor.

If you are looking for a sport, then tennis is a wonderful activity for all skill levels. It is wonderful for keeping the mind and the muscles sharp. Chess could be a fun hobby. It is a game with many rules and strategies to learn over a lifetime. This game can be played anywhere, at any time. I can see some good chess tournaments going on. Look around your community. What works best for your area? What works best for your friends and family? Do some research. Then go have fun!

Connect by being creative and changing things up with

different activities. Some activities are obvious. Going to see a movie, playing miniature golf, or eating out or going are all fun. However, not all activities have to cost money. Game night is always a hit. Get out your favorite board game or a deck cards. Restaurant at home is inexpensive, but fun to plan and execute. Plan with your friends what will be on the menu that night and cook the meal together. Be sure to set the ambiance with some music, candles, tablecloths, and table decorations. Be creative.

Make some popcorn and work on a large puzzle together. Or have a couple of different puzzles on the tables, then everyone can move from one project to the other as the evening goes on. Somehow our family always has lots of food involved in our activities (our family really likes to eat). So, be sure to plan and prepare fun snacks for this activity as well.

Be creative. You already have activities that you enjoy doing but shake it up sometimes. Find some events that are happening in your town. There are oftentimes free concerts and plays in our area. Everyone enjoys taking a blanket and picnic to sit and listen. Free is always a bonus!

If you are married or dating, please also take time for date nights. We all need time alone together to get away and have fun. It is important to connect outside of the routine of life. As our relationship grows and becomes closer all our relationships will be enriched. Make date nights together a priority. Everyone will benefit. Think about going on dates that you would have gone on when you first met. Did you go to movies? Bowling? Miniature golf? Concerts? Long walks? Dinner and dancing? Working out? Go do those things that you did at first. It will bring back some fun memories as well as rekindle some flames that might not be burning very brightly.

The other option is to do things you've always wanted to do

together. Have you wanted to take dance lessons together? Do it! Have you wanted to take a painting class together? Do it! Find some new and interesting activities that might shake some things up in your relationship.

Moms and dads, take your children out on dates as well. Our children consider this the greatest privilege in our house. Mom takes son, Dad takes daughter, Dad takes son, Mom takes daughter. Mix this up and let the children decide where they want to go and what they want to do. This gives one on one conversation with each child which eliminates competition for attention. These are some of the most relaxing and fun times we have with our children.

Take the child you are with out to dinner at their favorite restaurant (or maybe give them three options to choose from if you don't want to end up at your local fast-food joint). I have the best conversations with my children during these times. They feel free to open up to me when we are one on one. They also love getting to be the center of attention. I'm pretty sure that my children walk away from this time together feeling more loved than any other time. And, for me, I get a deeper insight into all that is going on in the heart of the child. Beautiful.

When our son was younger, he loved to play Uno with me on our dates. We always ended up at an ice cream shop in a competitive Uno tournament. Laughter was in abundance during this time. The older he got the more he won at Uno and the more he enjoyed our times alone. I'm not sure whether it is because he knew he could beat me or if he just liked our time together. Either one worked for me. I think it did for him too.

How about a vacation with some friends? Some of the most fun of vacations is planning. Get together with a friend or a group of friends and come up with a great vacation plan. Are you going to the beach, going skiing, visiting a historical site, or going camping?

Once you've picked what your vacation will be, start your planning by mapping out your route. Take some time to research what you might see along the way. Decide what your lodgings will be. What works best for your group? Hotel? Bed and Breakfast? RV? Think about food options. Will you be eating out? Cooking in the kitchen at the place you are staying? Plan all your meals together.

What activities will you be doing on your vacation? Plan these out but leave room for flexibility. Remember to leave room for time to rest. Even a short nap from time to time can help your vacation be more fun. Working through all these decisions can build your relationships, give each person a vested interest in the vacation, and learn valuable lessons together.

Big vacations can be great fun and wonderful bonding for you and your friends and family; however, keep in mind that you can also plan weekend trips or even day trips. Doing multiple of these each year will give the members of your group a deep sense of belonging.

The nice thing about day and weekend trips is that they can fit into all budgets. Going hiking for a day can be potentially free. Take meals along with you – you would have to eat whether you were at home or out on the trail. Find a train to ride. Visit a local museum to explore. Caverns are always fun.

Again, some of the greatest bonding will be over the planning of the event. Have fun and include everyone.

Are you looking to develop a deeper, healthier relationship with a specific person? What does that person enjoy?

Baseball? Dance? Art? Architecture? Maps? Wineries? Working out? Get involved in what they love. This doesn't have to take a lot of your time. If it is baseball, then you could watch Sports Center for a few minutes to be able to discuss the teams and players. Art? Then go to an art class together or visit a museum. You can buy books to learn some about what your friend loves. Ask them some questions. They may know more about the subject than you are aware. They might be able to teach you a great deal about their favorite subject. Show an interest and they will appreciate your time and effort.

Another way to connect with the people you love is to find ways to serve together. There are so many people in need. A neighbor down the street whose loved one just passed away, the hungry and homeless on the other side of town, the elderly who don't have any family members living nearby, the children on the other side of the world who need shoes. The opportunities to show love are endless.

Find out what interests the people in your circle. What do they have a heart for? This may be different for each person. This will make this step more interesting and will open our eyes to the diverse needs of others. Pick a different passion each week, each month or each quarter and plan how you will serve together.

Research the different opportunities in your area. Ask around. You may have some friends who are already serving in an area where you would find great joy and satisfaction. Some opportunities don't require an organization to work through. Loving on a family who is struggling financially by cooking a meal or going grocery shopping is a great way to bless others. Raking leaves in the yard of an elderly neighbor, mowing a lawn for family struggling with illness or doing some laundry for a mom who has recently had a baby are simple tasks that don't require a lot of time or energy.

Serving together can build strong bonds. Think of the people you have worked with on difficult tasks…there is a strong connection there. You will work side by side encouraging others and that will help you get to know one another better. The other benefit of this tip is that serving others in need helps put our own lives in perspective and will develop an attitude of thankfulness. We could all stand to be more thankful. Be blessed by blessing others.

What about sending mail to your friends and family members? Oh, the joy of getting snail mail! We all love to see our names handwritten by someone who loved us enough to take the time to send a note. This can work for you in so many ways. First, brainstorm together people you all think would enjoy getting a letter or card from you. Then just sit down and put some heartfelt words on paper.

Use your handwritten notes to let someone know how much you love and appreciate them. Be specific. The recipient will love and appreciate you for it. This is another opportunity to teach us to be more thankful, to think about people who invest in our lives or touch us in some fun or meaningful way.

We need to know we are special. We need to know that someone loves us. And, they take so little time!

Make this simple. Make this easy. The little things can make such a difference in your relationships. You can build bonds with simple ideas. Put just a little effort and time into these ideas and you will find your friends and family members feeling loved. Tackle one at a time. No need to implement all these ideas at the same time. You might end up feeling overwhelmed. See this as an investment in your future. Make small changes one at a time. May you enjoy beautiful times of encouragement, happiness, bonding and fun.

Write the ideas you have for connecting with others down in

your journal and start taking action today for making this happen.

Dream!

"Keep your eyes on the stars, and your feet on the ground."
Theodore Roosevelt

One of the common threads I have noticed in the lives of people who are dealing with unhealed emotions is the lack of ability to dream of wonderful futures. We need to dream to keep hope alive. If all we ever think of is the past, today, and the sorrow we are living in, then hope eventually will die. Then the downward spiral gets out of control.

So, what can we do? I think a great place to start is to think about what we dreamed of doing as children. I wanted to be a doctor when I was a young girl. Really, my heart was for helping people who were hurting. I never went to medical school, but the cool thing about what I'm doing now is getting to help people physically as well as emotionally. I have a deep passion for natural and integrative medicine and for seeing people healed in all areas of their lives. Studying natural health and sharing that knowledge is a joy to me. Getting to work with people one on one provides a deep sense of satisfaction. And, of course, I'm extremely passionate about the 28 Day Reframe book and seeing you healed in a profound way. Of course, I also have more ways to help people brewing in my head and heart. Doing these things that match my desires, passions and heart took a lot of dreaming and believing that I could help people. You must dream and believe!

Pull your journal out and start processing through your dreams.

Think about what you were excited about as a child. Did you want to be a fireman or police officer? Well, then what I know about you is that you have a heart to help people. Start thinking about what you can do to help people now. Did you want to be a singer? Then how can you get back into music? Start taking piano lessons? Maybe you can join a local choir. What about professional athlete? You could join an adult softball or basketball team, start biking, or find a group to walk with on a regular basis. What about those of you who wanted to be chefs? These days there are so many wonderful cooking classes at local grocery stores and at your local community college. I have friends who wanted to be interior decorators. They can also find classes at the local community college.

Did you want to be a lawyer? Get involved in your local CASA (Court Appointed Special Advocates) to help neglected and abused children making sure they don't get lost in the overburdened system or get stuck in group or foster homes that just aren't working for the child. It's a great way to be involved in the legal system as well as be a constant adult presence in the life of a child.

What about those of you who wanted to be a nurse? There are so many wonderful volunteering options available for you. The first idea that pops into my mind is nursing homes. There are so many lonely people in nursing homes who could use some tender-loving care. What an amazing difference you could make in their lives and no doubt there is so much you could learn from them!

Sportswriter? Sounds like a blog is in order. Teacher? There are so many volunteer opportunities where you can use that gift.

You can also take your passion as a child and start thinking about your next career. You are NEVER too old to follow your passion to some degree. You may not be able to be a professional athlete at 60, but you can find some way to be a part of the sport you love.

Start making a list of all the things you loved as a child and find some way to incorporate those things you still get excited about into your life today. You can think big and small here. Just find things you love! Going back to your childhood will show you what your innate passions are. As children we didn't have any presuppositions about what we were expected to do or required to do. So, going back to the beginning is a great place for us to start to find what we truly love and enjoy.

When you begin to do those things that you are passionate about, you begin to feel more alive. You begin to feel hopeful. When you begin to focus on the positive, joyful feelings you have, the negative will fall away.

I also want you to start dreaming about the future. What do you want to be doing five years from now? What about ten years from now? Really, please stop and think about this. You deserve a wonderful life and future. You deserve fun. You deserve joy, peace, and enjoyment. Don't just think about it, write it out. Putting this on paper makes it more real, right?

Start writing out what kinds of people you want in your life. We all deserve people who will support and encourage us. We deserve people who will help us be courageous and strong when we are feeling fearful and weak. We deserve people who will support our dreams, goals, and desires. So, who are those people?

Start writing out the career or business dreams you have. What can you see yourself achieving? What have you always wanted to do that you've never done? What about that business idea that you had? What about the book you always wanted to write? Just because you haven't done it before doesn't mean you can't do it now. Trust yourself enough to step out and do something for your future. Do it no matter what someone else thinks or says about it.

I don't remember really loving art as a child; however, I have found that I love finding ways to express myself creatively. Doing art with my daughter, encouraging her passion is what got me started in painting. Now, I don't paint for other people. I'm not interested in hanging my art in a gallery. I truly do it for the process. Maybe it's like running for some people. The process feels so good to me. Quilting is also something I have also found I really enjoy. For me it's about the creative process and the hand-quilting at the end of the process. Who knew? You see, I've been paying attention to what I really enjoy doing. Instead of just mindlessly going through life, I've stopped to pay attention to what is going on in my head and my heart when I participate in these activities.

What if you are in a position where doing something you are passionate about isn't possible? I meet people all the time who struggling with serious health issues. For some of them learning to rollerblade or even starting a garden are activities that are too physically demanding. So, begin by believing that you will one day (in the very near future) be able to do those things which you are not able to do today. Love yourself enough today to begin by preparing for the future (and having fun with the preparation).

Let's take gardening for instance. You love being out of doors. You love the idea of growing your own food (and sharing with friends and family). So, instead of spending your evenings watching TV, start doing research. There are a million gardening blogs out there. Obviously, the library has books in abundance. As you are researching, start planning and putting your thoughts and ideas down in a journal (or Word document). What kind of garden do you want to have? What do you want it to look like? What do you want to grow? When do you need to plant? When do you need to harvest?

Okay, so you get the point, right? Do the research you need to do as the prep work for all the fun you intend to have in the future. I don't know about you, but I also really love to do the research that is needed. So, it's a win, win, win. You get to dream and look forward to the future while you are having a great time prepping for that future. And, if you never get these things down on paper, then you will never have a plan.

Chalene Johnson said something that really has made a difference in how I've approached what I pursue day in a day out and how I pursue those things. She talks about goal setting in a new way in that her arrangement of priorities is unique. My takeaway from all she said was simple (because I'm a practical girl). Sit down and write some goals. Then you are going to categorize them. Are they career/money making goals, relationship goals, fitness/health goals, emotional goals? Now, what is your top priority from that list right now? Is your marriage struggling? Then your top priority better be to strengthen that relationship (yes, I know it takes two, but still make it your priority even if your spouse is not making it theirs). Are you struggling financially or in debt? Then your priority goal needs to be career/money making. Are you dealing with serious health challenges? Then your priority needs to be fitness and health. If you are feeling lonely, then your priority is to build and grow current relationships and well as develop new, healthy relationships. Now that you have determined what your focus needs to be for this period of time, make sure that each day you are doing two to three action points that will push you toward reaching that goal. Still find time for the other goals. It's not that they aren't important. It's that right now you have a priority, and you need to be focused on it.

Out of all that you have written down as you have dreamed, what is it that you really need to focus on right now? What are two things you can do today that will help you obtain what you are seeking? If you are reading this before bed, then put those things on your calendar to work on tomorrow. It can be as simple as sending a text to a friend. Maybe you need to make a healthy eating plan. Do you need to take steps toward the new business you want to start? Do this each day. Get these things down on the calendar. We are so busy these days and it is just too easy to let these things slip by. But, if they are on the calendar and we look at the calendar (or we get our calendar notices – yay for technology), then each of these action points are more likely to get done.

Personality Differences

I've observed something in my time living in a foreign country and spending time with people from other cultures. Americans have this idea of an "ideal person". This person is an early riser, courageous, not afraid of anything, extroverted, bold, outspoken, focused and perfectly dressed (I could go on and on, but you get the point). People from other countries don't seem to have the idea of what someone "should be". They tend to look at people as individuals with unique personality traits. They leave room for personality differences.

I've heard people from other countries and cultures say things like, "I am not very organized" or "I have a very sensitive personality" or "I am afraid of many things". In general, you aren't going to hear that come of out of the mouth of the average American, because those things just aren't tolerated or seen as very impressive in our culture. Now, if someone has been given a diagnosis such as ADD, then it is seen as perfectly acceptable, but have someone say that they frequently have their heads in the clouds, that they aren't organized or that they just can't seem to focus these days, well those are just seen as weaknesses. Showing a weakness seems to be taboo in our culture these days. But what if we all were able to share a small personality difference? Could we possibly become more tolerant of others if we did all share these differences?

I am an introvert. Now, I'm very social. I love spending time with people and enjoy it most in small settings, either one-on-one or with a handful of friends. However, put me in a large room with a large group of people whom I do not know, then most days I'm not going to feel very comfortable. There is the rare occasion when I get excited in a setting like this when I start to wonder who I'm going to meet and what opportunities will be presented. I've been told by people who later became my friends that they thought I was stuck up or that I was intimidating when they first met me. It really does just make me laugh when I hear that from people. I certainly don't feel stuck up nor do I ever intend to intimidate someone, but I understand how I can come across as aloof in a room full of people. Sometimes in large group settings, I'm already done emotionally from the beginning. I want to go home and refuel or just sit with a close friend and talk. So, I can imagine how that can come across as unfriendly. I've truly made an effort to push myself regardless of how I'm feeling in those types of situations. My hope is that the world will look at an introvert like me (and like those of you who are introverts) and instead of assuming that I'm stuck up they would assume that I'm an introvert and just want to having a deep conversation with someone I trust.

In her book, Quiet: The Power of Introverts in a World That Can't Stop Talking, Susan Cain does an amazing job of explaining introverts from the inside out. She also breaks down how introversion is not very well accepted in our culture. For those of you who are introverts (or if you live or work with an introvert), you'll love this book because she also explains how valuable introverts are in work, personal, and social settings. Cain can help you figure out how to use your introversion to your advantage.

What if we all looked at those personality differences as just differences and not necessarily weaknesses? What if introverts could look at extroverts and see the gifts that an extrovert brings to the table? What if a highly focused, type A personality could look at the more laid-back personality as valuable and even necessary? I think we'd make less assumptions about one another (and therefore have less conflict) and be able to forgive each other more quickly when we realize that we all just approach life differently based on our personalities.

So, let's start with ourselves, because we know we can't change anyone else. Start looking at your friends, coworkers, and family members as people with unique personalities, unique life experiences, and unique outlooks that make them who they are. These unique qualities mean that they bring different strengths to the table. Now, this also means that they bring personality traits that aren't our favorites (just like you and I do) that need to be overlooked sometimes. Let's try to consider that we are all beautiful, unique beings with gifts and talents (and challenges) and try to not beat one another up for those things that are different from us. Let's lead the way on this one and see what happens.

Affirmations

The purpose of an affirmation is to uproot and rewrite any ugly thoughts or words that have been planted in your head by family, friends, co-workers, the media, or any other sources. When someone says something to you that is negative you have a decision to make. Are you going to allow that negative input to be planted in your mind and heart where it will grow and choke out joy, life, and peace?

Whether those things are easy to fight or not usually depends on who says it, how it is said, how often it is said, and the ground that was cultivated in your mind prior to that. Some people say things that we can easily just brush off and move on. However, there are thoughts that get planted in our minds and hearts that are hard to fight off and challenging to uproot.

The amount of time and energy that it takes to uproot and rewrite ugly thoughts is the reason why I have become much more careful about the music I listen to, the movies and TV shows that I watch, and the people I spend my time with. My hope for you is that you will truly think through this so you can clean up your life. Do you want to listen to negative music and then have to spend time rewriting those negative thoughts? Movies can stick with you because they work so hard to evoke emotions with the volume, the music, the lighting, and the visuals. Having to spend time rewriting those thoughts and emotions is not what I want to spend my time doing.

We're going to have to live in this world and interact with family, friends, and co-workers. Some of those people are going to be unkind, so let's not add to it by being unkind to ourselves. Allowing unnecessary input into our lives is our being unkind to ourselves. Please stop it.

I know, we've touched on this earlier, but I just can't emphasize enough the importance of keeping your mind and heart protected. You wouldn't let crazy people into your home making it a mess, would you? It's the same with your mind. Be the gatekeeper. Don't let things in that don't serve to make your life better.

Okay, so now we have to uproot those ugly thoughts and build positive ones. Affirmations can serve you in this way. But again, it's not just about repetition. Choose to believe what you are saying. Smile when you say them. Make sure your tone is positive. I realize at first some of these will be a little hard for you to believe because you've been believing lies for so long. So, you'll have to fake it a little at the beginning. However, after you have said them for a while you won't be faking it. Sometimes you just have to convince yourself.

I love when people write their own affirmations to suit their situation, but I'm happy to provide you with some. These will serve you well.

Forgiveness

I choose to release all unforgiveness in my life. I choose to forgive and receive love. This love spills over into all areas of my life. I share that love with everyone I come in contact. Love flows in my direction as well which provides great joy and peace.

I lovingly forgive myself for anything I've done and all that I have not done. I rejoice in the ability to forgive and the freedom that comes as a result.

I lovingly forgive others for hurting me. I also choose to forgive others for the things they didn't do that I hoped they would do. I am grateful that I am able to forgive. I embrace the freedom that comes from all of this forgiveness.

I am worthy of forgiveness. I receive the forgiveness extended to me by others.

Today as I forgive, I give space for healing. I release all guilt, shame, condemnation, and fear. I receive acceptance, peace, love, and kindness.

Health

I take care of my body by eating healthy foods and exercising on a regular basis. I take care of my mind by filling it with only positive thoughts. I take care of my emotions by forgiving myself and others. Every day I make healthy choices.

I choose to have power over all sickness, disease, and pain. I choose life, health, and wellness. I am healed and completely whole.

Life flows now and forever.

I embrace healing. I embrace life and allow it to flow to every part of my body. Health, life, and healing are the building blocks of my path.

I want to be healthy and whole. I am healthy and whole. I deserve to be healthy and whole.

I grow stronger and stronger every day. Every part of my body, all the way down to my cells, grows stronger each and every day.

Every part of my body functions exactly the way it was meant to function.

I exercise regularly to stay fit, healthy, and strong. I love myself enough to put in the effort and invest the time. I deserve it!

Choosing food and drink for my body is easy. I only choose that which nourishes my body bringing life and health to all my cells.

My body was made to heal, so I choose that healing.

I pay attention to what my body is saying to me, and I invest my time, effort, and energy into bringing the very best to my body.

I breathe deeply bringing oxygen to every cell in my body.

I sleep deeply every night feeling rested each morning. My dreams are beautiful and encouraging filling me with peace and excitement for life.

Strength

I am strong and courageous! I can and will accomplish all that is ahead of me. I overcome all obstacles in my way.

Confidence empowers me to take action and live life to the fullest.

Feeling confident, assured, and strong is a normal part of my everyday life.

I choose to put positive thoughts in my mind and heart. I guard my eyes, ears, mind, and heart. I deserve to plant beauty in the garden of my mind. The beauty is life to my mind, body, soul, spirit, and emotions.

I am strong, confident, and full of enthusiasm.

I am fully dedicated to my personal growth, mentally, physically, emotionally, and spiritually.

I have the will and the desire to complete any project I put my mind to.

I have unbreakable confidence in myself, my abilities, and my perseverance.

I am confident, strong, and powerful.

I boldly go after all that I want in life.

Love

I am lovable and have an abundance of love to share with everyone I come in contact.

I deserve all the good and love that life has to offer.

I accept myself. I trust myself. I value myself. I love myself unconditionally.

I love others as they are and accept that I can only change myself.

Love is flowing all around me and flows in my direction.

Today I choose to love myself unconditionally.

I accept who I am to my core with complete and deep love.

I am happy with who I am and look forward to further growth and love in my life.

I deserve to be happy and to be loved.

Every single day it becomes easier to love and accept myself.

Today I choose to love myself unconditionally.

I accept who I am to my core with complete and deep love.

I am happy with who I am and look forward to further growth and love in my life.

I deserve to be happy and to be loved.

Every single day it becomes easier to love and accept myself.

Choosing Life

I choose to have a good attitude. I choose enthusiasm.

I am gifted and talented in unique ways. I choose to use those gifts and talents to bless the world. I assess my gifts and talents with kindness and excitement.

I work hard at all I do. I choose to do all my work with great integrity, honesty, and discipline.

I enjoy laughing and find humor in everyday events and interactions. I choose to not take myself too seriously and am able to laugh at myself when necessary.

I identify my goals easily and each day I work toward those goals. I choose to do something each and every day that gets me closer to achieving those goals.

I leave the past behind, choosing to learn from it and grow. I live in the present and work toward the future. My future is bright and full of joy.

I am adventurous and energetic. Connecting with others in those adventures brings love and joy.

Today I choose life to the fullest. I believe in myself and know that the best of my life begins today.

Beauty is all around me. I choose to see, experience, and acknowledge all the loveliness in creation.

In all life experiences, I choose to be 100% present, living with awareness and intentionality.

Each day I choose LIFE!

Interacting with others

I am a great listener. I show empathy and kindness to all whom I come in contact. I choose to be patient with my friends and family members.

My desire is to bless others with my words and actions. I take others into consideration when I'm choosing what I'm going to say and what I'm going to do.

I surround myself with friends and family who encourage me and build me up. I accept love and support from people who have great energy and positive words.

I look at all interactions with an objective eye, believing the best of those I love.

I choose to be a peacemaker which involves action and understanding.

Courtesy and kindness flow out of me easily. I see opportunities to bless others everywhere I go.

I allow others to bless me with their words and actions, seeing it as a beautiful opportunity to receive love.

Letting go of offenses is easy for me. I forgive quickly and allow myself to heal fully.

Deep, mutually rewarding relationships come my way and I am grateful for them.

Congratulations!

Here we are at the end of our time together. Know that I am immensely proud of you. You have done the work that no one could do for you. Healing seems to be a narrow path that few seek out, so count yourself as a fellow traveler with a small but powerful group of others who have done the hard work. I applaud you. I wish I could hug you in person and tell you how amazing you are for choosing this path and following through.

Please don't stop here. 28 Day Rebuild is the follow-up book to this one. It is just as practical and helpful. My hope is that you will do the work of building a life you hope to have. This will be a one brick at a time journey and a fun one at that. Again, this will be a challenge that I took up myself and have passed on to others.

Keep pursuing what is best for you – healing and growth. Stay open to love and relationships that are a blessing. Choose to be a blessing. Find ways to nourish yourself, physically, spiritually, mentally, and emotionally. Choose life. Choose JOY!

Blessings!